NIPPLES TO KNEECAPS –
TO DIE OR NOT TO DIE WITH CANCER

by Mandy Brown

Shoreline Publishing House
Devon, UK

This book is dedicated to all the people who face, or will face, a major challenge in their life that other people say is impossible to overcome.

It is written for people with cancer – past, present and future.

It is written in memory of my father, Charlie Hobbs, who always listened, supported me and most of all, believed in me. He was diagnosed with cancer, and passed away in 2012, at the age of 83.

It is written with gratitude to our children Alexander, Dean and Renate who grew up hearing "Believe in yourself and everything is possible" "A life lived in fear is a life half lived" and "You have a wonderful spirit inside you – let it shine!"

I hope our story and how we changed our life has a positive impact on you all.

Contents

Contents i

Prologue iv

What is *Nipples to Kneecaps – To Die or Not to Die with Cancer*? iv

Who is this book for? iv

Why did I wait to publish the book? v

What is my overall aim in writing *Nipples to Kneecaps*? v

Who were Mandy and Steve before the cancer diagnosis? vi

Chapter 1: The Death Sentence 1

Chapter 2: A Close Shave! 10

Chapter 3: Toilet Humour 18

Chapter 4: Can I Sign? 25

Chapter 5: My Vision 31

Chapter 6: Deluded or Focused? 38

Chapter 7: The Sales Team 42

Chapter 8: Proud Alexander 47

Chapter 9: New Game, New Shame 52

Chapter 10: Life in Their Hands 56

Chapter 11: Sick Bills 61

Chapter 12: Skating on Thin Ice 66

Chapter 13: Madder than Madeleines   73

Chapter 14: To War!   78

Chapter 15: Too Fragile for Sex!   84

Chapter 16: Another Nail in the Coffin   89

Chapter 17: Midnight call   93

Chapter 18: Deadliner   99

Chapter 19: Dying for Cold Turkey   104

Chapter 20: Feel the Fear and Do it Anyway   109

Chapter 21: Crypt Humour   115

Chapter 22: Skin the Fish   121

Chapter 23: Me and Mrs Melly   129

Chapter 24: Special Bond   134

Chapter 25: The Bell Tolls   138

Chapter 26: Foiled Again   144

Chapter 27: Following in His Footsteps?   150

Chapter 28: A Laugh a Minute   159

Chapter 29: Dark Opening   163

Chapter 30: Notes and Crosses   167

Chapter 31: The Walking Dead   174

Chapter 32: Final Countdown   178

Chapter 33: One Last Secret   180

Chapter 34: Flying High   186

Epilogue   190

What has happened post cancer? 190

What did we both learn from that experience and
episode in your lives? 194

Defeat Cancer PLAN 195

Appendix   200

The Healing Minute 200

Research Studies and Books 200

Epigenetics 200

Cells & Neuropeptides 203

Placebo 204

Laughter 205

Mindset 207

Meditation 207

Complementary/alternative practices 209

Nature 210

Jacuzzi of Despair 211

Comedies 1980s 212

Thanks   213

New Books Coming Soon by Mandy Brown   214

Contact   215

Prologue

What is *Nipples to Kneecaps – To Die or Not to Die with Cancer?*

It is a book of hope and inspiration. It is a true story about Steve who was diagnosed with terminal cancer in 1986 and sent home to die. He was given just three months to live. The story covers a two-year period of the most dramatic, funny and painful events that happened in the lives of Steve, his wife Mandy and their son Alex. Thirty years later, Steve is alive and well. What happened, what we did so differently compared to others at the time, and how he survived to this day is revealed in *Nipples to Kneecaps – To Die or Not to Die with Cancer*.

Who is this book for?

In 2015, Cancer Research UK predicted that one in two people in the UK will get cancer at some point in their lives. This book is for people who have cancer today, for those who are in remission and fear its return, and for those who may receive the diagnosis in the future. It is also for the family, friends and carers of those adults and children who have cancer or other devastating, potentially fatal diseases.

Why did I wait to publish the book?

Over the years, we have (as a family) shared Steve's story and, I believe, given hope and inspiration to all those who have heard it. However, I waited thirty years to publish *Nipples to Kneecaps* for the following three reasons.

1. Steve had three seemingly impossible goals to fulfil, which all involved a time factor – he has now achieved them.
2. Some people with cancer go into remission only to have it reappear five, seven, or even twelve years later. I wanted to make sure that Steve wasn't in 're-mission' but cured. I think a thirty-year run is long enough, don't you?
3. Last year, Steve finally *chose* to watch a film about cancer. Up until then he would always turn off any programmes related to hospitals, cancer wards or cancer patients.

What is my overall aim in writing *Nipples to Knee-caps*?

My overall aim is to give you, the reader, hope and in-spiration that you too can achieve the impossible.

Nipples to Kneecaps is an important story to be read and shared because if you find yourself facing your worst fear, your circumstances seem hopeless, or if you ever feel powerless, you can remind yourself of Steve's story and, as a result, feel empowered to change the predicted outcome – despite the odds and expectations of others.

I want you to understand that if you are suffering with ill health, or a doctor has diagnosed you with a progressive or terminal illness, you can change your prognosis.

I want to inspire you to find ways to make changes in your life today and to recognise how wonderful life is, even when you seem to lurch from one disaster to another.

If nothing else, I hope to touch your soul – that you may know me in your heart and draw strength from our story.

Who were Mandy and Steve before the cancer diagnosis?

The first time I met Steve's mates was at Russell's birthday party at Snobs nightclub in Birmingham. They greeted me with comments such as, "So *you* are the mystery girl!" "We were dying to meet you!" "Congratulations!"

A slightly inebriated Russell swung his arms around us and happily explained to me, "Steve here is real fussy. He's famous for only going out with a girl for one date, so we couldn't wait to meet…" He suddenly swirled us around attracting attention and shouted, "Mandy, the

vi

'special girl', who had managed to make it past more than one date!"

I was embarrassed but secretly pleased. Steve said to me later, "I just knew those other girls were not the *one*, so it wasn't fair to go on a second date." A typical matter-of-fact Steve response.

When we first met, Steve was training to be a chef at Birmingham College of Food and Domestic Arts so I only saw him at the weekends. I ran home from school every dinner time so I didn't miss Steve's phone call. There were no mobile phones back then. We spoke every evening on the phone and wrote love letters to each other every day.

Steve was the first to say 'love you'. He shouted it to me outside his mum and dad's house as I was driving off in my car. I was too shocked to reply.

When he finished college that year he moved in with my parents and me. We were just eighteen years old.

We were that sickening young couple who spent every moment together – holding hands, cuddling, planning our future lives. Some said it was unhealthy. Except for work hours, we were never apart. Our separate lives merged into one.

Steve did extra evening shifts as a wine waiter at The Grand and The Albany hotels in Birmingham so that we could save for a house. Mum and I would wait up for him to return. At three o'clock one morning, he arrived home in the taxi holding a champagne glass and a bottle. He'd been waiting on Diana Dors, Leslie Crowther and Arthur Askey (all famous household names at the time). "Diana asked me to sit and drink champagne with her," he said, "so, I saved a bottle for you!"

Most nights, Steve and I talked into the early hours. We discovered that we had so much in common, including the desire to do martial arts, and a love of dance music (especially the songs played on Radio Luxembourg). We also shared similar beliefs.

One such belief was that there is more to us than just flesh and blood. There are things that scientists can't explain, but we can sense, feel and postulate that they exist. The esoteric world fascinated us both. Our first field of interest was ley lines. As teenagers, we both experienced strange feelings in some places – as if 'picking up something not of this world'.

We discussed and questioned so much. Did we believe in astrology, palm reading, mediumship, ghosts, astral travel, herbalism, even witchcraft? What were talismans? What was the Kabbalah?

One of my brother's judo friends, Bryan, was a great source of occult knowledge. He was not like the others in the judo team. He had a silver-topped cane and wore a cravat and a silk-lined cloak. He drove a bright-red Morgan Plus 4 sports car. His idea of a first date was to book a ticket on the Orient Express. When my dad insinuated the date was 'excellent foreplay', he replied aghast, "No, Charlie, it was purely platonic!" Bryan was a certainly a gentleman with the ladies.

Bryan gave us some sage advice: "Whatever the topic or belief – do your research in depth, become a master of it – then, and only then, can you offer an opinion."

Steve and I explored how we felt about Jesus, God, Christianity and the many other religions. At that point, we considered that maybe all religions are the same in essence and connect to the same greater power – an incomprehensible, universal male-female creative source or energy.

I always knew that I was not just a brain and mass of chemicals in a body. I believed that we are eternal beings of some form, who live beyond the physical death. Steve trusted my instincts in that matter. He also had faith, even when I doubted it, in my ability to somehow tap into what we fondly called 'ooby-dooby stuff' – meaning anything paranormal, preternatural or metaphysical.

As children, we had both spent considerable time being alone – wandering through bluebell woods, watching dragonflies dance over shimmering lakes, paddling in meandering brooks and cloud spotting while lying down in dreamy meadows. We had both been content in our own company and in awe of the amazing, beautiful world in which we lived. Country bumpkins, perhaps?

As an eight year old, I played with imaginary friends in the trees. *We* would collect wild flowers and make headdresses from ivy. I told Steve about one of my strange habits: "I used to strip a twig and bend it into a loop. Then, holding both ends, I would scoop up and collect spider-webs from the privet hedges."

As an adult, I discovered that spider-webs have been used for wound dressings since the first century AD. I often said I should have been a surgeon, as another of my strange past times was dissecting dead insects, pinning their parts onto a board and labelling them! In later years, Steve became a microscopist for beekeepers. One day, while he was performing his microscopist duty, I phoned him. He greeted me with, "I can't talk yet – I'm in the middle of shaving the hairs off a bee!" So it seemed entomology was yet another of our shared interests.

Steve proposed to me one rainy day as we were sheltering in the Baroque archway of the Midlands Bank, in Wolverhampton. It was not a romantic, kneel down on one knee proposal; he simply held my hands and said, "We're meant to be together so we might as well get married." We bought the diamond ring that day from an antique shop.

When Reverent Merry said, "We only have the 1st of May left. It's not a popular day to get married as it's the pagan day of fertility," we both chorused in reply, "Sounds ideal to me!"

Getting a mortgage, however, in 1982 was a challenge – especially with interest rates around 18%. The Cheltenham & Gloucester advisor said that Steve earned far too little. We had already decided that we wouldn't include my future teacher's salary when applying for a mortgage. We wanted that as bonus income and to give us the option for me to stay at home when we had children. Steve didn't hesitate. "I will get a new job then! What's the point of me staying in catering if the pay's too low to give *us* what we want?"

Following this decision, I recall that we were watching *Hill Street Blues* on TV as Steve was thumbing through the *Exchange and Mart*. He sat up and pushed the magazine towards me. "This is full of weird stuff," he said, "Shall we buy this book by Joe Karbo?"

The Lazy Man's Way to Riches by Joe Karbo was the first book related to mindset that we ever purchased.

In the spring before our wedding, we stayed at a friend's sea-front house in Borth, Wales. We sat looking out at the golden sunset over the sea, the song *It Must Be Love* by Madness playing on the radio, and we filled in Steve's job application form for a job as a sales representative for Campbell's Soups.

"One day we will definitely live by the sea!" I said. And so we began to make plans for our perfect future together…

Chapter 1: The Death Sentence

"My dear girl, I have seen many a patient in my time and we cannot help Steve. At best, he has three months to live, but we shall make sure he dies as painlessly and peacefully as possible."

I did not expect this – the brutal finality of it, declaring the end of a young man's life. The all-knowing consultant leans forward, putting his wise hand on my shoulder as he says these words. They tear at my insides, gouge at my soul and stain my heart forever.

But in that moment my only emotion is anger.

***

Steve looks like a fragile twig left for compost. At six foot three, he weighs around seven stone, maybe less. He refuses to get on the scales again. His skin is in yellow mourning. His pain and suffering are unbearable. At twenty-five years old, his x-rays turned the radiographer's face ashen. Later, we hear that the doctors doubted his recovery from the operation, but no one would tell us.

"My stomach looks like a Cornish pasty," Steve complains.

Angie, our nurse friend, is also not impressed. Seeing the scar later she says, "Looks like an autopsy sew-up job!"

Doped up on morphine, Steve's pain racks his body.
How can anyone endure such agony? A month earlier at
our son's first Christmas, Steve said, "If it turns out to
be cancer I will give up. The pain is too much."
This was my call. Did I believe in Steve enough? Did I
know him enough to expect him to fight for his life
when the doctors and nurses had given up?

***

My rage returns as I mull over the consultant's words.
How dare he proclaim Steve's death sentence to me as
if he were some kind of God!
Mr Rogers's gravelly voice continues, "We had hoped it
was Hodgkin's – cancer of the lymph glands. We do
have some success in treating that."
I look up at him.
"Unfortunately, the tests show Steve has several malig-
nant secondary tumours in his stomach, below his kidney, and in his bowel."
I glare at him in defiance.
He continues, "We cannot find the primary tumour. So
it's impossible for us to treat."

At this point, something rooted deep within me rears up
and I hear my own voice – steady but determined.
"With all due respect, Mr Rogers, you may be a great
surgeon, but you are not a cancer specialist. I know
Steve. He can fight it. I want him to see the oncologist,
Dr Kitt."

Cups of tea arrive from nowhere, and the image of our son's happy face appears in my mind. I will not give up the fight.

Despite Mr Rogers's protests that Steve was 'full up with cancer' and, in his opinion, should be allowed to die peacefully, I remain steadfast and demand that second opinion from Dr Kitt. Jamie, a cancer survivor, had told me about Dr Kitt, his *own* oncologist, "He will keep treating you right up to the end," he said, and I knew he wasn't joking.

Shaking his head at the futility, Mr Rogers eventually gives in to me and agrees to set up an appointment with Dr Kitt.

My heels clack in a steady beat as I walk down the ward. Steve is surprised to see me. It isn't the prescribed visiting hours. He waits for me to speak. I falter, not sure where to start.

"They know what's wrong with you. Remember I mentioned Hodgkin's disease?"

Steve nods and stares at me with the eyes of a lost child. I have decided to be frank with him. He needs to know everything, but I refuse to bring up the three-month prognosis on the grounds that I simply did not believe it.

"Well, apparently it was always going to be some kind of tumour. But it's not Hodgkin's."

Steve interrupts, "Tumour? What do you mean?"

I'd asked the same question. "Cancer. You have a type of cancer."

Steve lays back in his bed. His stomach bloated out absurdly from his skeleton draped in flesh. His face is

3

gaunt and eyes hollow. I can only imagine what is going through his head in the few brief seconds before he speaks. He holds up three fingers.

Counting them down he says, "One, I want to live – to be with you. I want to grow old with you." My eyes fill up with reciprocating love.

"Two, I want to see my son all grown up." Alexander isn't even one, yet he will be a lion of strength for us both in the months ahead. "And three… I want to be a fencing champion!"

What? Where has that come from? Steve doesn't even fence! I tremble inside. Maybe I don't know Steve as well as I thought. Later, he will explain to me that he had fenced once when an Australian supply teacher had come to his secondary school. Steve hates mainstream sports like football and cricket. We both do martial arts and dance, but I have never heard him mention fencing before.

"Steve, I believe you *can* beat this."

In truth, Steve lacks confidence in his own abilities and skills. He confided to me once or twice, "I feel like I fail to make the grade. I'm not good enough, or clever enough compared to others…" I know how wrong this is, but I'm aware of the depth of his fear, how hard it is to dislodge. In an instant, I decide to turn this negative thinking on its head and take a gamble. If I was wrong, I would have to live with the consequences – forever. Steve's eyes search my face looking for hope. His breathing quickens and I imagine the 'self-doubt demon' sticking pins in him and laughing in his ear. Looking him straight in the eye, I say "Steve, if you beat this, then nothing in life will defeat you ever again.

This is the greatest challenge anyone can face; I believe you can do it."

I hand him a small framed picture. Now much faded, the picture shows a sunflower with the words 'If you believe in yourself anything is possible' written at the bottom. The same faded picture will hang in our house for many years as a reminder of this time.

Steve turns to me and says, "I had suspected the worst – either kidney failure or cancer. I'd stopped asking them what was wrong with me and what the test results said. They kept fobbing me off. The nurses used to come and play cards with me on the bed, let me make toast at any hour, then all of a sudden, after this last operation, they wouldn't look at me or talk to me properly." He had seen them whispering about him too. "I knew then, it was serious. I thought perhaps there was no hope and I was dying."

So, on this day I tell him everything and we make a pact.

Steve says, "OK, I'm listening and let's agree… if you don't cry, I won't cry." I sit on his bed, not once letting go of his fragile hand, his eyes never leaving my face. The words pour out of me as I pass onto Steve every-thing I know so far about his cancer, what has been done and what we can expect next. Finally, I fall silent. Steve's sigh hangs in the air. The clock ticks on relent-lessly.

I venture, "Do you remember Jamie from Wombourne, who had cancer and was given the last rites several times, but still survived?" Amazingly, Steve remembered him. "I've tracked him down and he's given me the name of his consultant. Jamie's coming to see you today. And Reg – he wants to come this afternoon too."

Steve greatly admires Reg, who attends the same Corinthian Gym in Wolverhampton as Steve and my dad. Reg is a sports physiotherapist. Two years ago the doctors diagnosed him with stomach cancer. He refused treatment against the doctors' advice. But armed with a positive mindset as his only weapon, he somehow fought it off.

Steve doesn't ask the dreaded question 'how long have they given me?'
My instinct tells me he really wants to know the diagnosis, not to die in ignorance.
"Easier to fight something I know about than to fight the unknown," he says. But, is he just saying what he feels *I* need to hear?
Before I leave, I tell him about Doctor Kitt and the arranged consultation. I want him to know there's hope, but even after telling him about Jamie's recovery I just feel so exhausted. We lapse into silence holding hands and simply looking at each other.

Steve glances at the clock, "What about Alex?"
"Mum's looking after him. Dad's waiting in the corridor. He wasn't allowed in with me."
My dad is a great listener. His touch, his glistening and distraught eyes – his presence communicated what words could not. I know I need my dad.

"I'm glad he is there for you," Steve says, hearing my thoughts.

For a month now, Steve has been too weak, too ill to get out of bed, but today he smiles, grabs my hand tightly, and somehow finds the strength to get out of bed! He wants to show me that that he will fight for his life. Tears threaten to roll down my face as he stands up. The nurses rush over, but Steve brushes them off. "Huh! I'm not fucking dead yet!" He huffs and turns to smirk at their shocked faces. Together we walk slowly to the door of the ward. As it opens, my dad looks up in astonishment. Steve jerks his head in the direction of the nurses joking "They're worried I'll catch my death of cold!" Dad and Steve grin at each other. At this moment I know I have my Steve back. He's going to fight this.

Three days later, Dr Kitt is standing at the end of Steve's bed, shaking his head. So much is riding on this but his presence is dark, foreboding even. He offers no small talk as he scans Steve's file, but I feel he will be honest and open with us.
"We can't identify the type of cancer you have because we can't find the primary. Any treatment would be a shot in the dark without that knowledge. You are so full of cancer that I really can't give you much hope at all." He holds his chin in his hand and stares at us. We said nothing. He picks up the notes and turns each page painstakingly. I don't know what it is he's looking for but I can tell he is intrigued, and I desperately want him to agree to at least try something, some treatment. The

7

ticking of the clock at the end of the ward intrudes the scene – each tick growing louder and louder.

Finally, Dr Kitt peers over his gold-rimmed glasses, "I could try you on a strong cocktail of chemotherapy but, I don't know." He shakes his head, "It's… guesswork with you. I could keep on trying different combinations of drugs but…" He shrugs, "All I can say is that if the cancer doesn't kill you, the chemo probably will."

In my head, I shouted 'We'll take it! We'll take the treatment.'

"So when do I start chemo?" Steve asks.

Dr Kitt replies, "Three months' time."

My world reels. Inside my head I scream 'But he hasn't got three months to wait! Shit, is that Mr Rogers right? No, no he can't be!' I haven't told Steve how long Mr Rogers has given him to live.

Steve is impatient, "Why can't I start it now? I need it now. Can't I start it sooner?"

Dr Kitt pauses, contemplating, "No. That eight-inch scar on your stomach needs time to heal. If we start chemo too early, the vomiting could burst your stitches and then the open wound would not heal." I know that chemo drugs are effectively poison to our bodies, designed to attack the fastest growing cells – the cancer cells first – but then what about the rest? His hair? I reached forward and stroked Steve's black curls.

"We will send you a letter," Dr Kitt barked as he walks away.

Steve lets out a gasp of air, "Dr Sinister there has the bedside manner of a mortician that's for sure!" It's such a relief to laugh. Thanks Steve. I love your humour.

That night I lay in bed planning. I decide to wait a month and then demand the first chemo appointment. I just have to make sure he starts the treatment before that deadline of three months.

Chapter 2: A Close Shave!

How did we get here? To a point where the thought of death never leaves us?

My mind wanders back over the previous year: my pregnancy and how elated we were to have our first child, Alex. We were so happy, and then it all started to change. I shiver as the muscle memory in my arms returns.

***

"Good morning sleepy head." I chirped, smiling at Alex as he lay still asleep in his cot. He was late waking. My hand dreamily trailed over his pale sky-blue wallpaper, tracing the white clouds on it. I had slept in this room when I was pregnant and had caught chicken pox from the children in my class. My hand stirred the wooden mobile hanging over him. I had made it from the tiny wooden toys we bought in Germany. Alex did not stir. I leant over the cot and stroked his face.

"No! No!" I snatched him out of his cocoon of patchwork blankets. His tiny body flopped in my arms, devoid of life or energy. I have no clear memory of the next hour – extreme fear and panic does that apparently. I do recall the doctor asking me later, "Where does your husband work?"

I stared backed at him speechless, knowing the answer but unable to respond – I remember thinking, how weird is that. Luckily, Jane, our neighbour who had driven me to the doctor's surgery, knew that Steve was a Crown Paints Rep.

Steve has never forgotten the events of that morning either; at 9.45 a.m. on 16th October 1985, he was in the Texas DIY store in Oldbury with Bob, his boss. They were checking the 'Misty Shape Emulsion' paint stock when they heard over the public address system, "Will the Crown Paints Rep, Steve Brown, please come to the office urgently!" As Steve did not have one of those newly invented, brick-sized mobile phones, our doctor's receptionist (his 'detective') had managed to track Steve down and get the message to him.

We spent the next few nights standing vigil over Alex's cot at Wordsley Hospital.
"He's a fighter. He will beat this!" I said repeatedly in an attempt to reassure us. The memory of Alex's scream from the lumbar puncture still haunted me.
"But meningitis! He is only six months old. Why is he not responding?" Steve had never looked as helpless as now... as he clutched and stroked Alex's tiny fingers in between his own giant thumb and forefinger. He would have done anything to take away tiny Alex's pain and suffering.
"He will be okay. I just know it!" I said.
Steve nodded as if he believed me.

Three days later the doctors confirmed that Alex was stable. We began to relax. I looked at Steve's bloodshot, strained eyes. Alex's illness was the first time I had ever really seen Steve under a lot of personal stress. To lighten the mood, I pointed out, "Your eyes look like vampire eyes."

11

"Charming!"
"I like vampires. They are sexy!"
"Ha, ha! It's lack of sleep."
Usually, whenever Steve's head hit the pillow that was
that. He was out for the count and snoring in seconds,
but this month he, like me, had not slept well.

After a few weeks it was confirmed that our little soldier had pulled through. Thankfully he had no long-
term damage of the kind so often associated with meningitis. All three of us returned home – shattered, but
relieved. We felt blessed to have our baby back. "There
must be a God or something!" I said.
Our celebrations were short lived, for then came another blow! On the same night that we returned home
from hospital with Alex – the night of 11th November –
Steve collapsed and I knew something was terribly
wrong. The ambulance blue-lighted Steve to the Royal
Hospital in Wolverhampton.

The nurse took his history – were all those niggling
problems connected I thought?
It was a continual joke that when I was pregnant with
Alex, it was Steve who kept going to the doctor with intermittent pains! Apparently he had a groin strain. I
think Steve was secretly proud when the doctor said, "I
suspect you're being too 'amorous' in the sex department, young man. You need to slow down lad and leave
off it a bit!"
I laughed when Steve told me as I was heavily pregnant
at that stage and obviously we were being gentle and
careful in that 'department'.

There had been other incidents at work when unexplained pain had overcome Steve, such as when he was at B&Q Stetchford Lane, in Birmingham. He was carrying some paint tins across the car park and had a sudden searing, breathtaking pain in his stomach. He clutched automatically at the pain site. The released paint tins hit the floor and exploded – splattering poppy-red paint all over his new black leather brogues and suit.

The doctor, that time, diagnosed a 'nervous stomach'. Steve was prescribed painkillers and antacids.

These odd 'collapses' in pain continued. The pain intensified and the episodes multiplied like bacteria in a petri dish. He couldn't sleep at night and pain became his constant companion.

One day in October, Steve woke up complaining that his fingers were sore and swollen. We identified numerous tiny inflamed cuts covering his fingers that had become infected overnight.

"I have no idea where they came from," Steve puzzled. We applied antiseptic cream.

Steve went off to work. Mid-morning, he called me, "I'm coming home! Those infected cuts are all over me now. I was at Asda Tipton having a coffee. People kept staring at me 'cause my lower lip was actually running with green ooze. Bloody disgusting… and it dripped onto my shirt!"

As each hour passed, Steve discovered more and more infected lesions all over his body. It was as if the tiniest,

13

previously invisible paper cut, nick or spot, was now infected and throbbing with poison.

"I can hardly bend my fingers now. My lip is agony. This is getting worse by the minute," he groaned.

By the time we got to A&E Steve's face was puffy too. Puss oozed from the various cuts, including those made by his early morning shave.

The doctor, clearly disturbed, surveyed Steve from a safe distance, the doorway in fact!

"You should have come in sooner! This must have been going on for several days."

"No," corrected Steve, "it started this morning."

As we continued to insist we were telling the truth, there was a perceptible change in atmosphere. Other doctors began gathering around, murmuring, each one of them now wearing protective gloves, masks and aprons. Blood samples were taken, but no explanation given.

We waited and tried to catch their whispers. A senior doctor arrived, also in full personal protective equipment.

Steve was not impressed, "They're all protected from this infection, what about you and Alex?"

Steve was given an injection of antibiotics.

"We're going to send your blood samples off for testing. It may take some time. In the meantime, I think it best you go home. Here, take these tablets. We will contact your GP with the results."

I felt there was something they were not telling us, but I was not brave enough to question further. It was only much later on that we realised what had been going through their minds. A new deadly disease had hit the National Health Service internal watch list; one we would all soon know about through TV adverts and warning campaigns in our schools and communities. It would rival cancer and spread fear throughout the world. We, however, were in the dark that day, yet in Steve's medical notes, a doctor scribbled '?AIDS?' All we knew was they could not seem to get us out of the hospital quick enough.

Steve's immune system responded to the medication. No one at the time questioned his low white blood cell count.

Trips to the doctor continued. Various doctors at various times suggested his intermittent pain was possibly due to a pulled ligament, a back problem or kidney stones.
"Better just man up and get on with it," said Steve.

Of course when Alex was admitted to Wordsley Hospital with meningitis our attention was entirely on him. When the life of your child is at risk, you can't think of anything else. However, 'the pain monster' had clearly not forgotten about Steve and 'he' was back with a pitchfork of vengeance!
So, here we were, on 11th November, back again in A&E giving the nurse Steve's medical history in hope of some answers this time.
"Back to more waiting around and hospital canteen for you." Steve managed to joke in between pain spasms.

I faked a smile and stroked his open palm. Steve always offered his palms for me to stroke when he needed relaxation.

The admissions staff suspected kidney stones again, or his appendix.

Two days later the hospital doctors concluded that Steve had a 'rumbling appendix' and with no sign of the pain subsiding, out came the scalpel. The surgeon suggested I returned home with Alex to get some rest as they would not operate until the following day. At midnight Alex woke me up, crying for his daddy. We found out later that this was the exact time his daddy, in fact, went into the operating theatre.

***

When I arrived the next morning Steve was already sitting up in bed, smiling. I remembered him visiting me in the maternity ward. Alex had jaundice so we had remained there for two weeks while he bathed under blue lights getting a tan!

In those days it was common practice to be shaved just prior to having a baby.

"Stop scratching. Looks like you've got fleas!" Steve teased me when my hair started to grow back.

Now the tables had turned! A young male nurse had done the deed. Steve explained,

"I couldn't believe it. Out came this razor and talcum powder. The nurse asked me to undo my pyjama buttons. I assumed he'd shave a small area around my stomach. I've not got a lot of chest hair but suddenly I had none! The bugger shaved them off! And then he continued downwards…"

Steve mimicked the nurse's suggestion,

"'You can help if you want by holding your *appendage* out the way when we get to that bit.' Bloody hell, now my manhood was in danger! When that embarrassing bit was over – I did not dare look – the guy carried on further down my thighs. He told me it was standard practice for my operation to be shaved 'Nipples to Kneecaps'!" Steve shook his head in disbelief.

"So that's why I was 'itching' to see you!"

Steve tutted at me and shook his head.

I took a sneaky look at his 'bald appendage', and giggled at the nurse's handiwork. Yes, not a strand of hair anywhere from his nipples to his kneecaps; my poor Steve looked like a plucked chicken!

Chapter 3: Toilet Humour

Steve had his appendix taken out and was allowed to return home a few days later. He looked terrible, bless him, and after a week he was still complaining of serious stomach pains. Psychosomatic? Had they left something inside him after the operation? The doctor prescribed more painkillers. Steve battled on, but I often saw him grip his stomach and hold his side indicating intense pain. Neither of us had experienced surgery prior to this year, so we did not really know what to expect after such an operation. Maybe this was normal and Steve was just being a wuss?

But, the pain marched on. Beads of perspiration collected on Steve's upper lip as he moved. I could feel him shaking when we held hands.
By early December Steve was too ill to go to work. The doctor came and gave him two weeks off, suggesting he had internal bruising or possibly an abscess.

A few days later another doctor was called in and volunteered the opinion it might be a hernia or maybe an infection. Yet more tablets. The 'pain monster' became cantankerous, causing Steve to curse and gasp.

It was no surprise then that Steve collapsed again. This time on 17th December he was admitted to New Cross Hospital where they were determined to get to the bottom of the problem. He was given a bed in the children's ward as the hospital was full; so full in fact that the entire ward had been assigned to adult men.

Mr Rogers declared that he had a plan, "We are taking you off all of your painkillers so we can identify where the pain is stemming from."

I watched helplessly as Steve's face contorted in agony during every conversation, the pain etching the wrong lines on his handsome face. The length of his hanging pyjama cord was increasing each day in proof of his shrinking waistline. Despite this, Steve stayed cheerful. He amused me with his stories – what he jokingly called the 'Soap Opera Drama on the Ward from Bed 101.'

There was the episode of the young macho guy, who came in with a 'football injury'. According to Steve, he had a swelling between his legs the size of a football. The poor chap, while playing football, had kicked the ball and turned, causing his own testicle to spin inside its sack. The result? A huge swelling that just grew and grew till he fell to the floor unconscious.
Waking up, post operation, he had grunted to Steve whose bed was opposite,
"I need the loo. Where is it mate?"
"Er, it's down the corridor that way, but I really don't think you should be getting up and walking around just yet. I'd ring the nurse and ask for a bottle to pee in if I were you."
"No thanks, bottles are for sissies," he sneered and pointed to Steve's.
"Please yourself," replied Steve.

The young guy clambered out of his bed and swaggered down the ward like John Wayne. All the other men watched, their heads turning in unison as they followed his progress.

"Wait for it…" Steve said in hushed and anxious tones. The football hero turned right to the toilet. He disappeared out of sight. Then: Smash, Bang, Clatter, Clatter, Thud! The footballer's screams of agony echoed down the ward. He had collapsed to the floor in a heap, but not before taking a tea trolley full of cups with him. There was a communal intake of breath and a sympathetic chorus of,

"Oooow!" from all the guys.

The nurses rushed passed to the rescue and bundled the poor wreck into a wheelchair. His head flopped to one side. A trail of blood followed behind him all the way back to the bed.

"Having opened up his stitches and fainted, the urine bottle is his new best friend!" said Steve with his boyish smirk.

Steve leaned over to beckon me closer. "See the old guy over there next to Neil? Well, last night he was ringing his bell, shouting for the nurses to come. He was having a real go at them for taking so long. Anyway, finally a nurse came, who then scuttled off to fetch the chair commode. She drew the curtain round his bed…"

Steve started to chuckle like a school kid as he continued with the story,

"Well, we heard her helping him to stand up and then get onto the commode. He let out a great sigh of relief and the biggest fart you can imagine. And then... and then... a huge steamy pile of shit appeared on the floor under the commode. The nurse had forgotten to put in the bucket, so he just shit on the floor. We were all in hysterics as all we could see, under the curtains, was his feet dangling off the commode and the big pile of poo!" Steve loved his 'toilet humour!'

It was not all laughs though.
"Bloody animal wallpaper everywhere!" Steve complained one visiting time.
I looked down at the telltale paint hiding in the creases of my skin on my forefinger and thumb – royal maroon, forest green, chocolate brown. I had nearly finished Alex's wall mural ready for him to move into his 'big boy room'. Today I had painted the flags on the castle turrets and put some hair detail on the animals at Snow White's feet. I was sure Steve would rave about it when he saw it.
"I've nearly finished the wall," I blurted out.
"What?" He was still pointing to the ward's animal print.
I winced inside. I am so selfish! I wondered then if the wallpaper on the ward was a daily reminder that he was missing out on the approach to his son's first Christmas.

As every day passed, Steve was clearly weakening and fading. Was no one going to help him? Alex and I even asked Santa Claus to make his daddy better.

21

On 20th December Alex woke up at 5.10 a.m. and shouted, "Da, da, da!" non-stop till it got light outside. He wanted his daddy home NOW.

"Alex, I want daddy home too, but he has to stay in hospital to get better." Inside I felt I was kidding myself and Alex. This nightmare seemed never ending. "I know you must be getting fed up with boring mummy but nanny and grandad will be over soon. We can go to the park and feed the ducks."

This was met with his relentless, "Da, da, da!"

I sat in the rocking chair and tried to comfort him by pointing to the alphabet wall picture I had made when pregnant. It had been my first sewing project. Each letter had a tactile picture or part that he could play with. Alex reached towards it. He pulled at the string of the balloon detaching it from its 'B' square.

"Yes, buh for balloon." My teacher instinct kicked in – this was one area in which I was confident.

But, Alex shook his head and exclaimed, "Da, da, da." He rubbed the sparkly star shape in the 'S' square and smiled at me, "Da, da, da."

I could feel tears beginning to surface. I missed Steve so much, "Yes, daddy is a star."

I put Alex back in his cot with some toys. I hoped he would settle back down, but Alex was on a mission. He was determined not to give up! For the next few hours he was either jumping up and down, singing "Da, da, da" at the top of his voice (while rocking his cot sides in time to his chant) or sitting down, ringing the bell on his Fisher Price Activity Centre and whispering, "Da, da, da. Da, da, da."

I felt so sad inside for him. I was not his daddy.

22

To my surprise and delight the spell-casting Alex, however, had his wish; his daddy was allowed home on
Christmas Eve. Steve was happy to spend time with us
but he knew that things were just getting worse and he
still did not know why.
"Take the painkillers," the nurse smiled weakly.
"Well I am sure I will be back soon."

On Christmas Day Steve barely moved, as the pain was
so overwhelming.
But, he still managed to smile as an extremely excited
Alex tore open his presents revealing an Action Man, a
Tonka Toy digger and a shiny black car transporter big
enough for him to lie on.

Before Christmas, Steve had insisted I go out and buy
myself some presents to unwrap from him on Christmas
Day.
"Oh, thank you for my Charlie perfume," I smiled.
"It's my favourite," he said. I had worn it the first time
we met and on our first date.
"And… a CD of romantic classics. Good choice
Steve!" I laughed as I knew this was not his choice of
music, "Yes, you old romantic, you!"
Steve was romantic but in a different way to the norm –
a better way. He would leave me little personal messages around the house, on my pillow or in my diary. I
always felt special when I found them. He never bought
greeting cards. Said they were a waste of money, but he
designed and made his own cards for me, which I treas-
ured. He did not do flashy candlelit dinners and rose

23

petals on the bed, but wherever we were – at home, in the street, at a conference – we held hands. He always put my wishes first, and he so believed in me and my dreams… like when I told him we had to learn sign language.

Chapter 4: Can I Sign?

As a child, every summer I visited my grandparents in Germany. My grandfather was deaf. When he spoke I could not understand his 'deaf voice'. It made me angry when my relatives said,
"Mandy, just nod when he talks. We don't understand what he is trying to say either, half the time."
I wanted to be able to communicate with my grandad, not just smile inanely, guess and nod. I tried to pick up on his body language, gestures and voice. He had not learned sign language as it was banned in Germany. I never understood why, but felt sure it would help. We developed an almost intuitive communication and I felt remarkably close to him.
I spent hours with him in his woodshed, watching him make slippers, wicker baskets or helping him with his rabbits, which he bred for food. He took me around the neighbouring farms and I saw how they valued his skills and showered him with cakes, beer and hugs.
I announced at around twelve years old, "I want to be a teacher of the deaf!" When I repeated this years later, my mum said, "It's so difficult. You need to be clever to do that."

After my A Levels I took a job as a trainee chartered surveyor. I was the first female that Allsop Sellers Estate Agents had taken on. I aced the exams and came top ahead of all my male colleagues. But, I still felt drawn to the deaf world. I decided to discover what being a teacher of the deaf might involve. I was shocked. It was 1979 and deaf children in the schools I visited in

the UK were being reprimanded for signing, told to sit
on their hands and forced to speak – I was appalled. It
felt inhumane. So wrong. It seemed so clear to me that
if the child was allowed to sign they would then have a
form of communication. The teacher could then build
up their English skills using sign language as the
bridge. At the very least the deaf child would learn to
read and write in English as a 'second language' even if
they never mastered clear speech. I needed to change
this, to help these children, to become a teacher of the
deaf. I knew I had to do this for my grandad, for me and
for future deaf children.

Steve and I enrolled on our first sign language course at
Lady Spencer Churchill College, London with Ruth
Roberts, Brenda Sutcliffe (both hearing) and Reverent
Tom Sutcliffe (deaf). I was hooked!

I applied to university to become a teacher.

Steve supported me, "If you want to be a teacher, do it.
You will be great. You are clever. Look at all those A's
you got in your school reports. You can do this if anyone can."

True, I did get top marks, but I worked hard for them
and I always felt I was not as naturally clever as the
others in the A stream. I was working class. My father
was a lorry driver and I spoke with a Wolverhampton
accent.

Yet, I was so convinced that I would get on the course
at university that I decided to hand in my notice even
before I'd had confirmation of a place.

"Mr Phillips is not going to be happy with you,"
frowned Miss Simmonds, the office manager. All the

girls in the office were scared of Mr Phillips. He came across as abrupt and cold. I had heard him raise his voice at many people. Now I feared it was my turn. I closed the door behind me, stood up straight and simply told him, "I am handing in my notice to become a teacher of the deaf!" I grimaced waiting for the tirade. He put down his pen. Silence. "No one in the office knows this," he said, "but I have a deaf son."
I was flabbergasted.
"You will make an excellent teacher of the deaf. I don't want to lose you, but go for it!" Tears of gratitude and surprise overwhelmed me. 'Small world' I thought.

The first teaching job I applied for was in a primary school with a deaf unit attached. The school had a strong oral policy, i.e. no sign language used. I sat opposite the headteacher.
"Am I allowed to use sign language in my class?"
"The children do not understand sign language so there is no point," she replied.
"But can I anyway? I will speak and sign at the same time."
I told Steve later, "I am not sure she even agreed, but I did not hear a definite 'no, you are forbidden to sign' so I am taking that as a 'yes'!"

My class had twenty hearing and ten deaf children. On the first day I walked in and raised my hands to sign. I spoke and slowly signed to them all, "Good morning. My name is Mrs Brown."

Well, I got their attention. There was a flurry of excitement, looks of confusion and frantic hand waving and signing by the deaf children.

"You can sign?" one child signed to me.

"You will get in trouble," another warned.

"Not allowed!"

"Headteacher will be angry."

They signed so fast.

I held up my hand to signal stop and signed back, "Slowly please. Mrs Brown is learning sign language. The headteacher told me you did not know how to sign. How did you all learn to sign?"

After furtive glances between them one girl signed back, "My parents are deaf. John's mum is deaf. We all learn sign language, but shh, it's a secret."

I was overjoyed and signed, "The headteacher said we are allowed to sign in my class. It's okay."

I soon realised that on the occasions when I only used spoken English with 'my' deaf children, our communication was limited. However, when I used speech and sign language it was far easier and led to more in-depth conversations and educational content. Now, our communication was limited only by *my* lack of knowledge of some of the signs *they* were using.

The day my class delivered the school assembly, we used our total communication method – meaning all of the children, deaf and hearing, stood at the front with me and signed as they spoke. We signed and sang 'I can sing a Rainbow'.

I told Steve, "When the assembly was over, the headteacher came over to me and with a stern face said,

'Mrs Brown my office!' I thought 'Oh no, I'm in trouble now and I'm still on probation.' She had agreed for me to sign in my class; she had *not* agreed to allow me to sign in front of the whole school."

"But the kids love you signing to them!" Steve defended me.

"She said to me, in that curt voice of hers, 'Mrs Brown you signed in assembly. However, I watched all the other deaf children. They never took their eyes off you. That was the first time we have not had to pull any deaf children out of assembly for misbehaving or inattention. Carry on! Carry on signing. I shall be watching your progress closely.'"

"That's great. So now what?" asked Steve.

"I keep signing. I have her backing now even if the other teachers do not approve."

Within the year the school had changed its policy from oral to total communication. This meant all the teachers had to go and learn sign language, if they wanted to keep their job. There was some opposition in the early days and I often felt unwelcome in the staff room, but Steve always said "Take no notice! You know you're doing the right thing." He was right. Inside I just knew it!

School and my deaf kids seemed so far away now. "I was thinking about school," I signed to Steve, "My maternity leave will soon be over and I will have to go back to work." I knew I would not. I could never leave Steve in this state.

Steve could barely lift his arms, but he managed to reply in sign language, "Happy Christmas!"

It's strange but I have no idea what I bought Steve that Christmas. Looking back presents were not important, people are.
He was extremely ill in the night.

Chapter 5: My Vision

"If they find out I have cancer, I will give up. This pain is too much," Steve confided quietly to me on New Year's Day. I pushed the thought away, but it haunted me because I knew that if I was in his position, I too would probably give up.

I looked across at Steve that day as he watched Alex and Ashleigh, our young nephew, playing. Despite his pain he managed to smile at them and offer encouraging words. The cousins had great fun battling on the floor with Ashleigh's Star Wars figures and Alex's Action Man. Steve was always so good with children. It was one of the things that first attracted me to him. Some years before, John (my boyfriend at the time) had brought Steve to our house. We had some visitors there, friends of my parents, who had a shy and bored young boy with them. John had stood awkwardly in the kitchen, while Steve confidently and happily introduced himself to everyone, then went off to spend time with the young boy. Within minutes they were chatting and giggling like best friends. I loved that about Steve. He could talk to anyone and magically put everyone at ease around him.

January started with Steve seeing another series of doctors and, after collapsing unconscious, they finally readmitted him into the Royal Hospital in Wolverhampton on 7th January for yet more tests. Another operation was planned, but before it took place he was, strangely I felt, allowed home overnight. Alex slept peacefully for

31

the first time in months that night. He did not wake till 5.45 a.m.! Steve, however, had to return early that morning to the hospital so as to prepare for a laparotomy. The consultant, Mr Rogers, explained to us, "The barium enema scan shows what look like fat lumps in your stomach glands. 'Pockets of something' can be seen all around your stomach and bowel area – fluid perhaps, leaking from your pancreas?" he mused.

On 21st January, they opened up Steve's 'not so old' appendix scar and took some samples of the suspect fat lumps.

On 23rd January, and thirteen stitches later, Mr Rogers phoned me asking me to come and see him. I wanted clarity and I was desperate to hear exactly what they had found. But, it was a brief meeting and though he mentioned Hodgkin's disease, he still would not commit himself to a diagnosis. And what was Hodgkin's disease anyway? There was no internet in those days so I couldn't research it myself. Until a firm conclusion was reached, which wouldn't happen until they had completed the examination of the cell cultures removed from Steve during the operation, no one was going to spend time explaining to us what all of this meant. So the marking of time began.

On autopilot, I returned home and opened the front door. I felt numb, but the sound of laughter from inside – Dad and Alex having fun together – pressed the 'play button' in my brain, allowing me to engage again with the world. I opened the lounge door slowly, trying to catch a sneaky glimpse of happiness. Alex was balanced on my dad's knee as my dad sang,

"This is the way the ladies ride.

Pace, pace, pace, pace, pace.

(Alex bounced up and down, wobbling from side to side)

This is the way the gentlemen ride.

Gallop-a-trot, gallop-a-trot, gallop-a-trot.

(Dad's knees moved faster and Alex's hair flew in the air)

This is the way the farmer men ride.

Hobble-de-hoy, hobble-de-hoy, hobble-de-hoy."

(Dad moved Alex from one knee to the other giving Alex a bumpy ride. Alex squealed in delight.)

My mum was nibbling the skin at the side of her fingernails and pacing up and down as if she was in a different world. She saw me, frowned and explained, "I was having a lie down in your bed. Alex jumped on the bed all excited, but when he discovered it was me under the covers and not Steve, he pulled this really sad face. I felt terrible for him."

Dad turned his head towards us, "His daddy will be home soon," he called over.

Mum huffed at him and continued, "It's okay for you, you got showered with kisses all day long!" Was this the way it might be? My dad taking the place of Steve? I shuddered and threw off the thought. One day at a time, Mandy, one day at a time.

The long awaited diagnosis day was due on 28th January – one day after my 24th birthday.

33

However, it was the night of 23rd January that I had my own earth-shattering and spiritual experience, which left me in no doubt as to the cause of all Steve's pain and what we had to do.

I lay once again in my bed – alone. I could hear Alex breathing gently through the intercom baby monitor. My bed, our bed, felt cold. I missed Steve's warm body. I longed for Steve. Every night he used to reach over and hold my hand as we slept or rest his hand on my leg if I turned onto my side. I missed him so much. I shivered. I just could not get warm. The room was tomb dark. I liked it dark, as I slept better, but Steve always wanted the landing light on which shone irritatingly into the room through the door, which he always like to leave open a little.

"I need the light on so I can see when I get up," he'd say accusingly. Steve frequently stubbed his toes or tripped over things when negotiating the darkness. (In later life Joyce, a close friend, referred to it as 'foot spooks.') Now though… it was pitch black.

I lay there and my mind wandered down its well-worn track – what if Steve was seriously ill this time? What could be wrong with him? He'd been in the hospital so many times now and they had found nothing 'big'. So what was it? Why did he keep collapsing in pain?

I felt a shift happen in the room as if someone had just come in.

"Nan?" I called into the darkness. She often visited me at night time when I was a child. She'd died when I was still small, but I'd felt her presence many times since.

As clear as anything, as I lay my head back down on the pillow, I heard her say three little words, "Steve has cancer."

So, it was final. These simple words rang true. I did not doubt them. I now knew it. Steve had cancer. With tears of frustration and fear, fighting back the awful truth, I began to cry, to sob, to howl. I cried till the early hours of the morning, seeing only bleakness and loneliness ahead for Alex and me.

The rays of sunshine forced their way under the curtain. My mind hadn't stopped and was still racing, my tears still trickling, but in those long hours I had made a decision. I suddenly stopped crying, sat up in bed and announced aloud to my bedroom walls how it would be from now on. A plan of action began to pour out of me – I was determined, exceptionally clear in my mind and totally focused.

"Okay, I am only crying for me – because I am scared of being left alone, without Steve," I chastised myself out loud. "Crying now serves no purpose at all. I will not wallow in self-pity. So stop it now! Steve needs me to be strong for him. I will cry if, and only if, he dies." I took a deep relaxing breath, "Crying is a waste of my energy. I will channel all that crying energy, all that

35

sadness, all that self-pity into something far more positive – into fighting for Steve, to keep him alive."

I still felt the 'invisible' spirit arm of comfort around
my shoulder. "Thanks nan for telling me. Thanks for
the heads-up… I think." I smiled. I could do this!
I knew now, for sure, that when I went into the hospital
to meet the doctors this is what they would tell me,
'cancer' would be their conclusion, but now I was also
determined that I would be prepared.

The plan of action formed in my mind. I would meet
the consultant. I would ask him for all the medical details, including the treatment options. I needed information – not sympathy or advice, just straightforward
truth – I needed the full information to help Steve get
better. And, Steve would be surrounded only by positive people holding and expressing positive thoughts.
Anyone else, and I mean anyone, who projected otherwise would be banned! We could beat this. I just had to
believe that with all my heart, soul and energy. It was
the only way. My mission was to find the positive in
every negative, to turn every negative into a positive
somehow. I had to be strong for the times when maybe
Steve would not be. The more I talked to myself in this
way the stronger I felt. It was as if the whole of the
spirit world was gathering around me, protecting me,
arming me with the weapon of 'positivity'.

I developed and wrote down a PLAN.
- Find Jamie from school, the one who had cancer.
  As far as I knew he had survived. If so, I needed to

know how. Steve would need to meet Jamie and people like him to learn how to fight this.

- Call Reg, our physiotherapist who had also been diagnosed with cancer, and refused medical treatment, but still lived. I remember his mantra 'mind over matter.'
- Arrange to see the consultant and insist on a clear and accurate diagnosis and treatment plan.
- Phone Steve's parents and get them to come to the meeting with the consultant. I felt they should be there as Steve was their son. My nan told me it was cancer, but they would need to be told by a doctor.
- No crying at all! None! Surround Steve with *only* positive, optimistic, happy people. Anyone who couldn't do this would be banned and have to stay away.

Thanks to the timely message of my nan I now knew what no doctor had been able or willing to tell me. Up to this point I believe we had all privately played with the idea it might be cancer, but more likely something was amiss with his kidneys, or some other curable disease of the bowels. At least I now knew it was cancer. What I did not know at that point was how advanced the cancer was and how far it had spread already.

Now I had a difficult phone call to make...

Chapter 6: Deluded or Focused?

"Hi, it's Mandy. You know Steve's been in and out of hospital for months now and just had another operation? I am meeting with his consultant, Mr Rogers, this Wednesday 28th for the results and wondered if you would like to come with me?"

Jean and Harry (Steve's parents) had not yet visited Steve in hospital although I had informed them every time he'd been admitted. I don't think they liked hospitals and I was sure they did not appreciate the seriousness of their son's condition. "I do not think it'll be very good news, so thought it best to ask you to come along."

I could sense Harry was taken aback, "Well Jean has a stamp meeting on Wednesday," he stammered. Jean had a passion for Russian stamps, was club secretary and had exhibited UK wide. Her displays were impressive and she was an encyclopaedia of information – her 'stamp' contacts even included the Prime Minster of India.

"Okay… but I really think you should be there for the results. Steve is in a bad way."

"Yes, of course, of course… okay. We will be there."

That Wednesday, Harry, Jean and I sat in the consulting room together when Mr Rogers delivered the blow giving Steve the three-month death sentence. Despite the 'three months' part being a shock to me, I surged into action calmly, asking questions and assertively demanding that second opinion from Dr Kitt. I sensed those around me thinking, 'How can she do this? Does she realise what has happened? That Steve is going to die?' Little did they know that unseen forces had warned me.

Jean stood up and Harry rushed over to her. The nurse took them both to one side. Behind me I was aware of a blur of activity. I could hear Jean crying softly as the nurse handed her a cup of tea. Harry standing motionless and silent beside her. I just continued my onslaught regardless. I was not going to give up until the consultant agreed to arrange for Dr Kitt to see Steve. His parents must have thought me cold or uncaring of their feelings. I was not. Maybe they thought me stupid to go against this doctor's professional opinion, but I was fully aware at that moment that Steve was relying on me to fight for him.

I believe Steve's parents, Mr Rogers, the nurses, our friends and family all thought I was naive and in denial of what they saw as the obvious truth. Steve was a frail walking skeleton, a mere shadow of his former self, in great pain and near death. I was on a futile mission to save him and they pitied me.

***

The following is a conversation I did not hear about until well over two years had passed since the medical consultant had passed judgement on, and dealt the 'death card' for Steve.

While mulling over the traumatic previous years, my mum finally confessed to me, "You know I went to Angie?"

"Why, when?"

"I thought you had cracked under the strain of Steve being diagnosed, so I went to Angie and asked her what she thought about you?"

"Really?" I was surprised and a little intrigued what Angie, a great friend and nurse had replied.

"It was that time when you were being so over the top, so super positive that I thought you'd gone mad. I thought you should have been in floods of tears and facing the worst and I told Angie so, but Angie said 'No, Mandy is one very strong woman and far from cracking.' She said we should all do as you asked." Mum shrugged her shoulders and quietly said, "So I did."

I felt really thankful to Angie for her quiet vote of confidence in me. As mum shared this tale of support, I remembered telling both my own mum and Steve's nan that they could not visit us until they could be in a room with Steve without blubbering all over him.

"I am sorry I had to ban you from seeing Steve, but you know why, don't you?" I asked.

"Yes, you were right. I felt so sorry for him and little Alex. I was concerned for you, but did not know how to help or what I could do – it was so sad, devastating and unfair," Mum explained.

We sat in the silence of our own thoughts, each replaying those early days.

40

Mum nodded, "But, I understand now… Steve only wanted and needed to have happy visitors, not people crying all around him. It really helped him."
I smiled as I remembered Steve's actual words, "I don't want miserable bastards around me!"

As I write this today I feel so thankful to both Angie and my mum. You understood me on a deep level even though, on the surface, perhaps my behaviour was challenging, uncompromising and maybe a little mad. You followed my wishes. Your strength in holding back the tears helped Steve too. Everybody was so compliant even though I am sure a few thought I had 'lost the plot' with the stress. But, I knew that in those moments I was actually the strongest I had ever been. I had my goal, my plan, my purpose. I had an unshakeable belief that this was our destiny – Steve's and mine – to get through this and be together. There was no 'we will beat this *or* … ' *Or* was not an option. Yes, there would be times when even I was rattled, but I'll come to that later.

On 28th January, we were all shocked when the USA space shuttle *Challenger* exploded on take-off killing its seven passengers. A sad day, made even sadder by the fact that today was the day I told Steve he had terminal cancer.

Chapter 7: The Sales Team

"Hi, Mandy. It's Bob from Crown Paints. How's he doing?"

"We're waiting to see the oncologist and hopefully get some treatment started. He seems happier in himself now he has the diagnosis. He has something to fight against now."

"So where did they say the cancer was?"

In that split second, I wondered if I should reveal the full extent of what we knew, but Bob seemed level headed enough. He was Steve's immediate boss at work and Steve had always spoken highly of him. Surely I could gamble on him working with me?

"They found secondary tumours or cancer in his stomach, bowel and right kidney. They can't find the primary, but basically, his torso is full of cancer." This devastating diagnosis tripped off my tongue almost glibly.

"Oh!" came his shocked response.

I must stop doing that. I should be gentler with people I chided myself.

Silence.

"So, anyway," I continued, "he is definitely up for visitors. Can you make it? One condition though – no sympathy or sadness talk. He wants to hear what's happening in the world, he wants to have a laugh and see smiles."

"Well yeah, of course," he stammered, "Well me and the lads were thinking of paying a visit, but we did not realise how serious it was… maybe best we leave it?"

"I know he would love to see you and the guys. Have a laugh!" I was waiting fingers crossed.
"If you're sure?"
"Yes, of course."

Bob and Jeremy sauntered onto the ward both in their pinstripe suits and broad red ties. Steve beamed at them in greeting.
"Still lazing around?" teased Bob. With this comment I knew that I could leave Steve in their care.
"I'm going to pop to the café for a bite to eat. Leave all you lads together. Behave yourselves!"

They were just leaving as I came back through the ward doors. I stopped to watch. There was lots of shoulder slapping, cheerfulness, what looked like an upbeat goodbye.
"See you guys!" shouted Steve to their backs.
As they approached me I could see the struggle on their faces to keep composure. They briefly looked back for a final wave.
I turned to accompany them out.

"My God. He looks terrible. I am so sorry, Mandy," Bob shook his head. His face crumpled as his eyes welled up. Jeremy's mouth was held taut and he stared at the ground.
"Thank you for coming and cheering him up. It really is appreciated."
Before, if I saw someone start crying, it would set me off like one of Pavlov's dogs. But, ever since the pact

43

that Steve and I made, my promise held and I did not cry.

They both nodded solemnly.

"I'll let you know when he comes out of hospital. Maybe you can visit again?"

Their eyes shot up to my face. I could read their doubt, their belief that he would never leave hospital alive, let alone come home. I was getting used to this involuntary response from visitors. I smiled encouragingly. Bob recovered quickly. Maybe it's a salesman's skill – the ability to hide their true thoughts and feelings? He reached over to hug me in support. "Yeah, we will look forward to it."

I then saw another exchange of knowing looks between them. This time with a little spark of unexpressed humour. Was he debating whether to say something cheeky, to cheer me up? For a moment they reminded me of naughty school boys. Yes, I could understand why Steve liked them – I sensed they shared the same dry and facetious humour. It made me smile.

"I will call you, Bob. Thanks again, Jeremy, for coming."

Steve was sitting up in bed. He seemed brighter. The visit had done him good.

He was holding an A4 booklet in his hand. I recognised the cover and logo. It was one of the *Crown Paints Monthly Review* documents. Not exactly thrilling reading but at least Bob was keeping Steve up to date.

"So, Bob gave you some work to do?" I gestured to the booklet.

Steve just smiled and patted the bed so I could sit beside him. The nurses didn't like it when visitors sat on the beds, but Steve would just laugh and tell visitors to ignore them. I snuggled up next to Steve. He opened the booklet, saying, "Want to see what's happening in the exciting world of paint and wallpaper? Figures from last month?"

I registered a glint of delight in his eyes as he scanned my face for a reaction. At the best of times it was hard to get excited about paint sales, but I was prepared to play along. As he opened the cover, I automatically made the BSL sign for 'my jaw dropped'. He roared with laughter at my stunned expression and sign. Inside the cover of this particular *Crown Paints Monthly Review* was glued the latest edition of *Razzle* – a porn magazine! What could I say? In a sense it was the perfect gift.

Being Steve, he couldn't resist sending ripples of shock and embarrassment around the ward, sharing his 'sales performance' with other unsuspecting patients. Frankly, I doubt he looked at the content too closely – he just liked the opportunity to spread some hilarity. In fact, we both enjoyed seeing the looks of confusion and merriment as that booklet did the rounds. It was a cut above the *Radio Times* and a bag of grapes.

45

Shortly after this visit from Bob, I received a call from Crown Paints head office. They modified the rules for us. I was so grateful. The tawny 1600 Vauxhall Cavalier was a perk of Steve's job, but they gave me full use of the car for as long as we needed and even sent someone round to fit a car seat in it for Alex.

"Isn't that great Steve?"

"Yeah… can't believe Alex is already in a car seat," Steve said, squeezing my hand with unsaid meaning.

Chapter 8: Proud Alexander

As Alex got stronger and more active by the day, I watched his dad, 'my' Steve, get weaker. It was almost as if some karmic exchange was taking place; but I wanted both my boys to survive. I would catch Steve looking at Alex with a strange glazed expression. I could sense his emotional pain and hurt that Alex might grow up without him.

In response to prompts of, "Are you okay?" Steve was able to flick that invisible switch to 'smile' mode and say with conviction, "Yeah, fine, fine."

My dad was great with Alex, but sensitive to Steve's feelings. He and I would talk about Steve's physical weakness and how not being able to play with Alex, as other dads did with their sons, must be difficult. The early days of childhood are irreplaceable.

Steve passed each day lying in bed or on the sofa, drifting in and out of consciousness as the morphine took a greater hold on him. He ate barely enough to feed a rabbit let alone a six-foot plus man – the effort of swallowing was too exhausting. Forcing himself to keep his eyes open he was clinging on to life, but missing most of it. Alex passed his days charging around in his baby walker, making surprise attacks on my impressive forest-like ferns. I would often catch him with a half-chewed fern leaf hanging from his mouth. He would loudly demand each mealtime with incomprehensible noises shouted at increasingly higher volume. Alex set out to make each day a new adventure of discovery, capturing any visitor in his play world, and melting my dad's heart in the process. My dad doted on his grand-children; he would do anything for them.

My dad was constantly at hand – helping with all the chores, lifting and carrying Alex for me and supporting Steve physically. Just being there as this strong male figure in our life meant so much.

Then one day, we realised what was actually happening. We should have expected it, planned for it, but it caught us by surprise. It was only a word but it nearly made our lives crumble. Time definitely stopped for a moment.

Alex, now 10 months old and toddling about already, came charging into the lounge. Alex was such a deter-mined little soul. All his energy had gone into making strides in this world and to get to where he wanted. Consequently, it was not until he was over one year of age, that he finally turned his attention from walking to talking. And what a day of mixed emotion that was!

In his hand Alex clutched another object we'd hidden from him and yet he'd found – my car keys! Steve chuckled at his son's skill. Alex, proud to show off his acquisition, held it in the air for all to see. Then he pro-claimed loud and clear, "Daddy!" as he thrust the keys into his *grandad's* hand.

Silence fell on the room. The penny dropped. It was my fault. I was always calling out to my 'dad' in front of Alex. He heard me saying, 'dad' or 'daddy' all day long, but to *my* dad, not his!

My dad's face was ashen, "Steve, I am so, so sorry. I didn't mean to…" he said with tears in his eyes.

"No, it's fine. To be expected. He sees you as his dad anyway – you are there for him. Honestly, it is not a problem." But the sadness in Steve's voice was tangible. "I couldn't wish for a better dad for Alex than you, Charlie."

Steve was imagining a future for Alex without him being there; it was unbearable for me.

I was determined that 'Grandad' would be the next word Alex learned!

Oblivious to the grenade he had just thrown, Alex turned his attention to his other toys. He clambered onto his favourite toy – his beloved sit-on Thomas the Tank Engine – and scooted into the hallway. It sounded like old metal roller skates rattling on the wooden floorboards. Steve shut his eyes. 'Grandad' and I grabbed the opportunity to escape into the kitchen for that typically English 'cure for all' remedy – a cup of tea.

***

Jamie and Reg, the only two cancer survivors I knew, were marvellous. They both kept in contact after visiting Steve that first day in the hospital, when they had shared their journey and fighting tactics with him.

Steve enjoyed repeating Jamie's story to our doubting friends, "We know this guy Jamie. He was dying of cancer. Jamie comes from a Catholic family so when it got near the end, they called in the priest to administer

49

the last rites." Steve paused to take in the atmosphere of dread. "The priest was waving his hand in the sign of the cross over Jamie and mumbling away in Latin when Jamie opened an eye and shouted, 'Oi, you bastards I'm not dead yet!'"

Steve laughed at their disbelieving faces, "Jamie had the last rites said over him three times… and he is still alive today, three years later!"

***

Time was ticking on and I began ringing Dr Kitt's secretary, urging her to arrange an appointment for Steve's first chemo treatment. "Please tell him Steve is feeling much better. He wants to get it started as soon as possible. His stitches are nearly all out now." I pleaded.

The direct approach paid off. We were rewarded with an appointment for admission just two months and two weeks after the dreaded 'death sentence' had been passed. I felt elated and then sick with foreboding. I had won the first battle – within the three-month deadline! I just hoped Steve would see it that way.

'Grandad' and I supported Steve as he climbed slowly down the stairs to Deansley ward in the Royal Hospital in Wolverhampton. It was located in the basement of the old Victorian building. Steve took one look at it and gave it the nickname it deserved, 'The Crypt'. I am sure it must have had windows, but I cannot remember any. It felt like a dungeon.

"Looks like something out of a sci-fi movie," said Steve as the nurse hung up the chemo drip, which was wrapped in foil. Was the foil protecting the contents, or us from the contents I wondered?

Steve lay on the bed for three days and nights as the poison slowly dripped into his veins. The vomiting started almost immediately.

Driving Steve home, I kept looking at him. What had we done? What had I done? He looked worse and weaker than ever. Steve was given three weeks off the drugs, to recuperate between cycles, but he would still be vomiting and suffering intense pain; when the three weeks were up he would have to return for another three days' treatment, continuing this cycle of torture until when, until what?... Dr Kitt's words pecked at my brain, "If the cancer doesn't kill him, the chemo will."

That night, as Steve sat retching and moaning in pain, I began to broaden my campaign. It was time to recruit the help of others. To every person who phoned me that night and to anyone I spoke to thereafter, I said, "Can you please ask everyone you know – of all and any denomination – to pray for Steve or to send him their positive healing thoughts?" I figured, what harm could that do?

Chapter 9: New Game, New Shame

That first month of chemo felt as if we were on a small inflatable dingy being tossed about by freak waves in a raging storm of pain, vomit and helplessness, with no sight of land.

Steve was being continually drained by pain in his torso. Alex, of course, was unaware of his dad's frail condition, and sitting still beside him was never an option for 'Alex the little explorer'. Alex would climb up Steve's body, trampling on his stitched-up stomach, while jumping in excitement to show his new toy to Steve's nose! Steve would 'grin and bear it' – these precious moments overriding all the negatives.

However, one day Alex was in for a shock. My dad had gone out to empty the bins, while I was in the kitchen washing out Steve's sick bowls. Seizing the opportunity, Alex crawled over to Steve who was slumped on the settee, half awake and no doubt trying to control the pain. The little explorer levered himself up and then found his climbing foothold on his dad's bony hips. Alex reached up to Steve's face, giggling. I heard a yell from Steve, and a genuine cry of terror from Alex.

As I walked in it took me a minute to understand what had happened. Steve, by now, was stifling laughter, but Alex's face was a picture – he wore the expression of an angry cabbage patch doll – all scrunched up. His eyes darted back and forth between Steve's face and the unexpected bounty he now had safely clutched in his little hand – a hank of Steve's jet-black wavy hair. Even though Steve's hair was his target, I must assume he hadn't planned on pulling it out, and he seemed genuinely shocked.

However, this instant of surprise soon passed and Alex realised he had an even funnier, albeit unique game to play – the 'Pull Out All of Daddy's Hair Game'. It was great fun, apparently, but we just knew that the next victim would not have such an easy time, if Alex attempted the same trick! At least the chemo seemed to be doing what it should (with a little help from Alex).

Steve decided he wanted a shower. Such a simple everyday routine was now a much bigger deal than you might think. I am only 5 foot 2 inches in height and Steve over a foot taller. Despite this, I would have to support and almost carry him up to the bathroom, then climb with him into the bath where I would hold him upright while he showered. As usual, we laughed our way through it – Steve making silly noises and comments, while I tried not to fold up in a fit of giggles and drop him. My strong, tall, dark handsome man was little more than a hunched up bag of bones these days, but he could still make me laugh; the real Steve was still undoubtedly in residence.

"Oi, watch out for my sexy, twiglet legs on that step!" he joked. This was usually followed by his impression of frog calls, "Ribbet, ribbet!" just to make me laugh as I struggled to keep him upright, walking in the direction of the bathroom.

We made it to the shower. Little did I know what horror lay ahead for me. I am not one of those people who is frightened by the sight of blood, panics in an emergency or transforms into a startled rabbit if shocked by something. But it seems I do have a phobia – one of which, until that day, I was blissfully unaware.

Steve sighed as the warm shower caressed his aching limbs. I held onto him, enjoying the physical contact (so rare in those days). I shut my eyes and savoured the moment of closeness, as the warm water fell over and around our naked bodies. But then something felt wrong. I felt my body tense. What was it? Something visceral and deeply unpleasant, that I couldn't put a name to. I opened my eyes and, instinctively, let go of Steve in panic.

"Urgh – horrid! Hate it!" I stuttered, shuddered and began retching. Steve wobbled, clutched at the shower curtain, but then steadied himself against the wall. His legs shook with the force of trying to hold himself up. "Sorry Steve… it's the HAIR… I don't like it. It's sticking to me." I scrubbed at my body in a futile attempt to release me of the wet strands that stuck to my body like superglue. "Urgh!" I whined.
Steve looked at me, nodding as confusion turned to understanding. "Ah, I see – it's *my* hair!"

I felt so stupid, so uncaring, so ashamed of myself. Here I was worrying about a few strands of clinging wet hair, while my husband was, well, barely alive. I felt pathetic, but I just couldn't help it! Even looking at the hair clinging to the bath sides made me shudder and retch. What a time to discover a phobia!

Steve's reaction to losing his hair like this? "Hair today, gone tomorrow!"
"I so love you," I laugh, "You can always make me laugh, even in *Hair Phobia-ville!*"

Laughter is definitely a medicine that lifts my spirits. I need it to build up my reserves. Pushing away sadness was a constant battle, so moments like these, that we manage to turn into 'comedy routines', definitely help.

***

Early in that first month after chemo an old friend from university, Louise, rang me. She had heard about Steve's cancer from a friend of a friend.

"You go and see Louise. Catch up. See the new baby. I'll be okay for a few hours," Steve encouraged me. I knew what he was thinking: he wanted me to have the support of friends just in case... Louise now lived about two miles from us so I felt it would be okay; I could get back quickly if I was needed.

Chapter 10: Life in Their Hands

I knew immediately something was off when I walked into Louise's house, even though Louise herself looked great. On the surface, she hadn't changed in the two years since I last saw her, but something was different. I scanned the room and my eyes fell on the baby photos.

Louise caught my look, "He died."

What? I did not know what to say or how to handle this. We had lost touch after teacher training college, but I'd heard she was pregnant. Doreen (a kind, loving lady who recently visited us to do some 'hands-on healing' for Steve) turned out to be a neighbour of Louise's parents. It was through Doreen that Louise had made contact again. 'Small world' I thought, but no one had said anything about the baby dying. I was unprepared. I felt guilty. On the phone we had chatted briefly about Steve's illness; Doreen had shared the news with her and I assumed that Louise was reaching out to me, as a friend, in this awful time. She had met Steve before we got married. When we spoke on the phone I'd said 'I hear you had a baby?' In reply she told me his name, Thomas, but said nothing further. I can only guess that it was too hard for her to explain over the telephone – the harrowing fact of her loss. Naturally, I'd assumed all was well. Why hadn't anyone warned me?

"I am so sorry." I spluttered out.

Tears welled up in her eyes. I moved over to hug her and I started to cry too. We sat suspended in time, just hugging each other. I was glad I had come alone leaving Alex at home with my parents and Steve.

"When I was pregnant I had a scan and the consultant said my pelvis was tiny. He said it would be best to book me in for a caesarean."
I listened, feeling my soul reaching out in sympathy to her. Poor, poor girl.
"But I went into premature labour. I told the doctor in maternity that I needed a caesarean. He disagreed and said I'd be fine."

Louise wiped her eyes and pulled away. I felt the surge of anger coming from her now tense body, "He was wrong. The baby was too big. I kept crying and telling the midwife that my GP had said I had a big baby and he would have to be delivered by caesarean. Well, hours later the doctor tried to use forceps, but they couldn't get my baby out. He was just too big and I was too small. Finally, I was rushed in for an emergency section. Afterwards they gave him to me and I held him. He was gorgeous, Mandy. He was perfect and strong looking. A big, healthy baby. I was exhausted, but happy. But, within minutes the midwife took him away to the neonatal ward 'for examination' she said. Terry and I waited and waited for them to bring him back.

The doctor arrived without our boy. He explained that our baby was in intensive care. Due to the traumatic birth he was now on oxygen and needed further tests. I was so scared and desperately wanted to see and hold him. I could not believe what was happening.

The hospital priest came to see us and asked if we wanted to christen him – normal practice for babies in a condition such as ours. It was surreal. We gathered round his cot the following day and he was named Thomas. The photograph on the mantelpiece is Thomas at one day old."

She passed me her cherished photo. He looked so healthy and so much bigger than my own son had been at that age. I handed it back, fearful of the next part of the story.

"The doctor told us that Thomas was brain damaged. During the birth, he was deprived of oxygen. Thomas was hooked up to life support machines to help him breathe.

The doctor said, 'It is unlikely he will ever be able to breathe on his own. Even if we could keep him on ma-chines for life we do not think he will ever be able to move or talk. The damage is just too severe. I am so sorry.' The machine would be switched off to spare him that, but we had a choice still. 'When we turn off the machine, you can stay here with your husband and we'll take care of him 'til it's over. Or you can come into the room and hold him in your arms till he… dies.'"

"Terry couldn't do it. He couldn't stay. It was just too much for him. He won't even talk about it now, but I knew my decision."

I waited, hardly breathing.

"Mandy, I picked him up. He was so lovely. I held him in my arms. He never did take a breath on his own, but I felt him go. It was peaceful. He died in my arms and I will never forget him."

Tears flowed down our cheeks. I felt distraught, but nothing compared to the pain that Louise felt.

Sadly, there was worse to come. After about five months, Louise's GP said it was safe to try for another baby. They did, but each pregnancy test came back negative. On further investigation, it was discovered that the traumatic birth had damaged Louise and she would never be able to bear another child. Such a terrible, sad story. My worries about Steve paled into insignificance. At least he was still with me, still alive. We had each other. We had our healthy baby.

I looked into her eyes and felt our souls instantly connect – no words were necessary.

"Doreen, my mum's neighbour, really helped me come to terms with what had happened," Louise continued. "I went to the Spiritualist Church – the healing helped me. I believe I will meet Thomas again one day and that my grandad is looking after him in spirit. That's how I found out about Steve."

"Oh, what do you mean?"

"On Sundays, they read out all the names of the people who need healing. I heard the name Steve Brown, so I asked Doreen if it was the Steve Brown who you married. She said yes it was. So I called you. I had to tell you how much they helped me."

Louise was so brave. Would she ever be the same person again? No, of course not. Many would have fallen into despair and a life of depression and lost hope. But, Louise was an inspiration. She went onto travel, live and work in many different countries, and to make a huge difference to other children's lives by being a great teacher. I am so grateful to Louise for thinking of me and reaching out when she did. It made such a difference, and I learned something really important from her about the strength and kindness of the human spirit.

Chapter 11: Sick Bills

"How are we going to pay the bills?" Steve asked.
He could not work, and if the doctors had their prognosis correct, he would never be returning to work. I was still on maternity leave and there was no way I could go back to work and leave Steve's side. I just had to stay with him as each minute was precious, and while I didn't accept that he would die, that bloody clock was ticking relentlessly away, taunting me, as if to say 'Tick-tock, time's a passing – let's see who's right'. Each new day reminded me that we were that much closer to Steve's inevitable death, according to Mr Rogers's Calendar of Doom, but also each day encouraged me that Steve had survived yet another 24 hours.

But what about the mortgage, and all the other bills we couldn't afford to pay? Walking through the hospital corridor one afternoon I passed a door marked Hospital Social Worker. Of course! They must deal with situations similar to ours every week. They will know how the benefits system works; how people like us can get help when disaster strikes. I walked in on the spur of the moment and introduced myself to a friendly young man who was really helpful. He made an arrangement for a home visit.

On the day of the visit some friends popped in – little did I know how important that coincidence was, as if someone was looking out for me. We knew Sharon and Mike from antenatal classes. Steve and Mike had shared the same humour; so were in fits of stifled

laughter during many of the presentations, but especially the one that showed a vintage
bath-time video. In it, a 'modern dad' demonstrated how to safely bath junior. It was a black and white production, straight out of the 60s. Consequently, the voice-over was in clipped BBC English, making everything sound like a wartime public information film, even when the 'modern dad' was simply bathing his son. Worryingly, the modern dad drooled "Oh I do love to get my hands on his firm little body!" We all spluttered. That phrase has passed into legend and to this day we repeat it at the most inappropriate times.

I hadn't remembered but Sharon was a social worker before she'd given up work to have her baby. So when the young man from the hospital arrived, she offered to sit in with me as a second set of ears. I accepted gratefully, as I was really tired that day. Steve and Mike 'babysat' the kids in the lounge.

The young social worker began talking me through the various benefit forms. He assured me, "Steve will qualify under the special rules for the terminally ill, due to the nature of his condition, the severity of the cancer. They process things quickly for people with fatal illnesses." That was meant as good news, I suppose, but I resented his assumption. I corrected him with a sigh and in my head I counter-attacked with 'Steve is getting stronger each day!' Sharon was silent throughout, but I was aware that she was squirming to the edge of her seat. I threw her a questioning look of 'what's wrong?'

The young advisor continued rabbiting on with his 'shopping list' of things to check.

He asked, "Do you have any life insurance policies?"

"Yes, we have something we took out with the mortgage," I replied.

"I suggest you arrange to cash that in straight away to give you some extra funds."

Sharon sprang up from her seat, outraged.

"Mandy, do no such thing!" She turned and addressed the startled young man, "*You* are a disgrace. What is your name? I am a social worker and the advice you are giving is completely inappropriate, and dangerous!"

I sat back as she tore into him. I began to feel sorry for him as he hung his head and tried to apologise, but she was having none of it.

"You cannot tell someone whose husband is seriously ill that she should cash in their life insurance policies. If Steve's prognosis is correct and they have no life insurance, because of your advice, that will leave his wife and child not only penniless, but homeless too!"

Bless him. He scuttled out looking so ashamed, and promising to get the correct forms sorted out as soon as possible. Sharon was so horrified though, she decided to follow up with a complaint. Although I never saw the letter she wrote it certainly had a remarkable effect. Several weeks later I received a phone call from the hospital social work team. The manager was offering to make amends and get us more assistance than we were actually entitled to. Every cloud has a silver lining!

I couldn't believe my luck. Suzie, our 'home help' (as they used to be called), came two mornings a week to clean the house and do the ironing. It was bliss to be given that freedom to use time in a way that pleased me, whatever I chose to do with it: whether I sat and played with Alex (who loved the extra attention); or massaged Steve's aching back; or even sat down at the piano and continued with my efforts to learn how to play. When I plonked away on the piano it really helped me switch off – probably because I had to concentrate so hard to get a recognisable tune! I loved my walnut piano – she let me escape and have fun.

As the weeks went on the number of the hospital sick bowls increased. There was now one in every room. We played loud, upbeat music throughout the house. Michael Jackson's 'Beat It' was a particular favourite, followed by Sting's 'Every Breath You Take'. Steve's music choices were deliberate. They added to our mission of all around positivity and keeping optimistic at all times.

"Alex, let's decorate daddy's sick bowls," I suggested, one day. And, thus was born a regular family activity. Steve chose various pictures – cars, castles, VW camper vans, which he meticulously glued onto his collection of plastic sick bowls and then covered in sellotape to protect them. Alex used his favourite stickers of the Care Bears and Transformers. Once completed, he proudly presented them to his daddy. What did I choose? Hearts, smiley faces and rainbows, of course!

I had an idea. "Each and every time you vomit, we will both say 'Look there goes some more of the cancer!'"

"Well, I have got to get it out of me somehow," Steve agreed and added, "Every time I take a shit, throw up, pee or perspire I could visualise some more of the cancer being ejected from my body, and good riddance to it!"

Thereafter choruses of, "Oh, there goes some more of the cancer!" rang through our house daily.

Chapter 12: Skating on Thin Ice

Leslie gave me my first proper job as a sales assistant after school and at weekends. I must have been around 13 or 14 at the time when I first started helping her out.

During the summer holidays Leslie asked me to babysit her children – Dawn and the new baby Kylie. Owning and running three ladies' clothes shops meant she had great demands on her time, and I was happy for the extra money and responsibility. I felt decidedly grown up!

Dawn was adorable but the original messy monster. Her play room looked like it had been in the path of a tornado, but I made a game out of putting it all back together again, tidying everything away, much to her mum's delight.

On one occasion when I was babysitting, Kylie had diarrhoea. The mess was so bad I just couldn't clean her up and was worried she was getting sore. I called her mum out of teenage desperation, and she told me to fill up the bath with warm water. I had never bathed a baby before. Come to think of it, Kylie was the first baby I had ever held. Somewhat apprehensively I lowered the poo-smeared Kylie into the water. All hell broke loose as the warm water provoked yet another bowel movement! Streaks of poo now floated in the water, swirling and gaining ground on her 'firm little body'! Should I pull her out? No – not clean yet, and still pooing! Should I leave her in? No – as she was getting even more covered in slimy poo! I began to panic, dipping

her in and out of the water like a pink marshmallow in a
chocolate fondue. What was I doing! Retching, I tried
to avoid the rivers of swirling poo as I plunged my hand
in the water to release the plug. Not my finest hour.
But, it's amazing what you can do when you have to!

Surprisingly, Leslie did invite me to baby sit for her
again! And, it was she who introduced me to ice skating. She also introduced me to Janet Sawbridge MBE,
the triple gold medallist for Great Britain in figure skating and ice dancing. I had gone along with Leslie and
Dawn to Solihull ice rink for Dawn to have some extra
private tuition from Janet. But, so fascinated was I with
what I saw that I started to use my wages to pay for my
own skating lessons with Janet.

A few months later, Leslie helped me encourage my
dad to come along and watch me in my first skating
competition. Until this point it was just a hobby and I
did not want to trouble my dad. I had seen how much
time he had spent ferrying around my brother, Geoff, to
all his judo competitions (he became British champion)
and, anyway, Leslie was happy to give me a lift. But
I'm so glad he did come to this event.

I didn't win a place on the podium that night but Janet's
father, who was watching from the side of the rink,
called my dad aside and told him 'Mandy has talent';
apparently Janet saw me as a 'young lady with promise'
– not as a solo figure skater but as an ice dancer. It was
so unexpected – I had never done any ice dancing before – and I was so proud that my dad was there to hear

67

that. It wasn't too long before I was selected for coaching and paired up with a young man who was to become my partner on the ice.

I had no idea what was coming my way. This new found passion of mine turned my life on its head, and all of my family became involved too. We were suddenly thrust into the world of ice dancing: local and national competitions, travelling to far-flung parts of the country, practising every day, both early morning and late at night.

School work fitted around our coaches' programme. I recall studying for my exams, sitting on a plastic, red, moulded chair in the café of Silver Blades ice rink, Birmingham. When the rink got too busy I simply opened my books and revised – despite the background of blaring organ music, kids shouting and teenagers pushing and shoving each other, larking around.

Those years taught me how to persevere even when progress felt slow, to pick myself up when I fell down – literally and figuratively; how to focus (even with hundreds of screaming kids hurtling uncontrollably around you); to push myself with a goal in mind. However, I am aware that due to the choices I made that I fell short of competing at the top, of not achieving my goal to represent Britain in the Olympics. But, I did meet those who had succeeded.

Wearing one of Janet's cocktail dresses (as I had nothing suitable to wear having turned up for a training weekend with only my skating dresses and PJs in my bag), I recall feeling self-conscious but privileged when she took me with her to attend a reception in the Birmingham Council Chamber for Olympic and World Champion John Curry OBE. While warming up for another competition at Bristol Ice Rink I met Robin Cousins, another Olympian and three times world medallist. I still smile at the memory of him shouting, "Mandy, duck!" as he jumped over my head doing one of his famous split jumps. And, when Janet moved our dance training to Nottingham Ice Rink, I trained alongside the amazing and soon to be famous Olympic and World Champions – Christopher Dean and Jane Torvill. My small claim to fame is that I remember being asked to show Jane how to do a lay back. This is where the lady bends backwards so her head touches the ice while skating at speed. I feel honoured to have met them and so pleased that I was able to introduce Steve to them at a skaters' party.

I realise now that I was surrounded by focused, disciplined people who wanted to win! I have Leslie and certainly, my parents and brother to thank for encouraging, enabling and creating that experience as part of my growing up.

Steve, bizarrely, believes he saw me skating in Birmingham when he was one of those 'teenagers larking about'. He said, "I fancied you then, but you were too fast to catch."

A year later we met properly. The guy who introduced us was, in fact, someone I knew from my skating circle of friends. These days Steve often reminds me, with a suggestive smile on his face, "I always liked to see you in your sexy skating skirts!"

***

"That was Leslie on the phone, you know, from skating days? She's heard about your cancer and is coming to visit us."
I was pleased. I had not seen her for some time, but I knew Dawn was now helping her mum as manager in the shop.

Leslie arrived with her arms full, carrying a huge basket of fruit. It was a wonderful gift. In keeping with most of our friends, she also offered to pray for Steve. We thanked her for this but it was noticeable how she kept turning the focus of the conversation back to what you might call a 'religious' theme. It appeared that she was excessively concerned about us both. In the years since we had last spoken, Leslie had taken up a new faith. She was now a Born Again Christian.

All this evangelical stuff was new to us. We had our own shared beliefs about religion, spirits, and the universe, formed in those long hours of talking all night as young lovers. I had also recently asked for prayers and positive thoughts from whoever offered. But, in response to Leslie sharing her religious viewpoint, Steve launched a rhetorical inquisition,
"So, you are saying that I have to accept Jesus will save me or I will go to Hell? When did Born Again Christians come about? Was it 1960s, 70s? What happened to all the young men in the First World War, who went over the top? The 16, 17, 18 year olds? I can't accept, 'Well they are in Hell!'" He continued on another tack,

"Ok, all the Buddhists? All the Japanese martial artists and those who follow Shinto… all in Hell? If that's where they are, I have more in common with them!"

Leslie was composed, as she did not mean to upset us. She had the best intentions. Before she left, we agreed to consider two things.

Firstly, would Steve attend a special healing service at her church, so that the congregation could pray for the cancer to leave his body? We had misgivings but we agreed. What harm could it do? After all, we reasoned, all healing energy comes from the same source and we were grateful for all the prayers offered on Steve's behalf. From observing the special service, I could see many parallels to other healing services we had attended.

Secondly, she left us to ponder the possibility that if Steve died any time soon, he would go to Hell, for not accepting Jesus Christ as his saviour. It was clear to us that she wanted to see us both 'saved' and that the healing service was step one in that process. However, then, as now, I struggle to comprehend how a compassionate, loving God would only accept into Heaven those who had accepted Jesus, sending the rest to an eternity of Hell. Isn't spiritual love unconditional? My spiritual encounters had always led me to feel that way. I believe, in essence, we all come and return to the same 'place'; we are all connected, all learning and it's a shame that mankind, with its various religions and practices, argues so much about the details.

I respect the right of everyone to choose their own spiritual path, whether evangelical or otherwise, and I certainly still hold much affection for Leslie, but the irony of the situation was not lost on me: a Christian comes to offer the fruit of temptation, with the message 'Hell awaits you'.

Chapter 13: Madder than Madeleines

"Thanks, Paul. Back to reality now!" I said.

I heard him sigh in response as I put my key in the lock of our oak front door. Laughter echoed down the hallway.

I put my squash racket and bag down, as we exchanged puzzled glances.

"Not what I expected," I said.

"I can only hear Angie's laugh," Paul replied.

Angie was an experienced nurse and a brilliant friend. She volunteered to look after Steve and babysit Alex so I could go and smash a squash ball around the court with her husband. It gave me some valuable down time; you can't worry about cancer and the future when there's a tiny rubber ball ricocheting towards your head at fifty miles an hour!

Paul and Angie were there when we needed them. Ironically, she knew and had nursed Jamie when he had 'terminal' cancer. She worked with the surgeon Mr Rogers, the same man who had given us Steve's death sentence. Although she never said so at the time, I later found out that she agreed with Mr Rogers's prognosis and feared Steve would never recover. She had seen how seriously ill he was and just couldn't imagine how he could get through it. She didn't want to let me down as a friend though and continued to support me all the way in being positive and encouraging. It was people like Angie that really made the difference. I doubt I could have done it on my own.

I opened the door, slowly taking in the scene before me. Angie was rolling on the floor, holding her stomach, tears of laughter streaming down her face.

"What's going on?" I could tell that the hilarity had got the better of them. They were in fits of giggles and just couldn't stop.

Steve was clutching his belly, cursing as he laughed while Angie rolled around on the floor, clearly having lost the plot, shouting, "Stop, stop, it hurts to keep laughing!"

"Bloody hurts you? What do you think it's doing to me?" Steve retorted.

Angie rolled over again, shrieking, tears flowing freely, "Sorry but it's... so funny!"

"Call yourself a bloody nurse!" Steve shouted.

"Okay, let us in on the joke," Paul butted in, shaking his head at his wife and rolling his eyes at me.

Angie looked up at Paul, then pointed at Steve, as if to say 'it's all his fault'. Laughter erupted again.

Finally, Angie pulled herself upright saying, "Okay. If I don't look at him I can explain."

We waited.

"Steve asked me to make him some Madeleines, in the microwave."

I interrupted, "Madeleines – coconut cakes?"

"Yes. I said I'd make them for him even if he only keeps them down for five minutes! I was in the kitchen making them and Steve sat here watching TV. Then I hear the little voice pleading pathetically, 'Ange, Ange. Come here. I think my hot water bottle's burst.'"

Steve never went far without his hot water bottle strapped across his stomach to ease the pain.
"I came in to have a look."

Steve took over the story, at this point, as Angie once again started to giggle. With mock indignation, he described the scene.
"Miss Professional Nurse here took away my trusty hot water bottle – so clearly leaking. She starts to help me get off my wet pyjama top when I notice that it is not the hot water bottle that's leaking, but 'me' – my stitches had burst! Instead of sympathising with me when I start to panic 'nursey' here just says, 'Oh, pull yourself together man!' then proceeds to roll around the floor laughing at her own joke. Meanwhile I'm desperately trying to hold my insides in, which is pretty difficult when I'm laughing too."

I rushed over to examine Steve's stomach through his fingers. I could see his insides. I reeled back in disgust and panic. Steve's eight-inch long scar had indeed burst!
"Oh my God, Angie. What do we do?"
I gawked at them both – expecting any moment for them to come to their senses.
"This is serious," I announced, my voice betraying my feelings. Inwardly I start to blame myself, thinking 'Oh no, this is my fault. I should not have left Steve. I'm forcing him to 'survive' when his body is just not up to the job'. Just as Dr Kitt had said, he needed to recover from the surgery, but oh no, Mandy was impatient, insistent, wanted her own selfish way. Now the chemo

poisons were racing through his body, killing everything in sight, not even allowing the surgical wound to
heal. How would his skin knit back together now?

I remembered my cousin Sonja having surgery on her
spine some years previously, but her body rejected the
metal plates. She was in constant pain and would not
heal. She had holes in her back which had to be packed
daily with fresh gauze to replace the puss-drenched one
from the previous day. The experience was agonizing
and frightening. Would Steve now have a similar fate?
All because I was too scared, too impatient, to wait the
full three months. It was my doing. I'd persuaded the
doctor to start early despite his own better judgement.
Selfish, selfish, selfish.

It was obvious that neither a plaster nor even a bandage
was going to repair this.
"We need to tape it together for now." Calmness returned to Angie's voice as she rummaged through our
first-aid box, "Nothing here strong enough."
Paul put his finger in the air, and rushed outside shouting, "Be right back."

He handed Angie a roll of bright-blue electrician's tape
from his van. She put a clean gauze over the gaping,
oozing hole, and with Steve pushing either side of the
'sunk' hole as close together as possible, she secured it
in place with the electrician's tape.
"That should hold until we can find out what needs doing next," she smiled.

The district nurse arrived the next morning. I listened intently as she explained the new daily regime of unpacking the gauze, the scraping of the raw hole in Steve's stomach, the repacking with gauze and liquid paraffin.

Finally, silence.

I glanced at her and Steve's expectant faces.

"Sorry," I muttered, "No, I think it's best if you come in to do this, not me. Can you?" She nodded and I left the room. I picked up Alex and cried softly into his dark hair – our secret.

Chapter 14: To War!

"Fuck off!"

I had always hated swearing. I could not recall my parents or brother swearing in my company as I grew up. Yet, here I was, pleased to hear Steve swear. Why? Behind those words lay an emotion, a force so strong that a human cell could react. Did I believe that – really? Did Steve believe that?

Every day the loud cries of, "Fuck off!" would be heard from the bedroom. Steve was barking orders to his body again, or truth be known, giving encouragement to the army of soldiers he'd created whose sole purpose was to advance, attack and destroy the enemy – the cancer cells that were in his body – the enemy within.

Steve needed to take back control of the inside of his body. He couldn't cut it open and rip the cancer out physically – despite the gaping wound in his belly – so he used the power of his mind to plan the campaign. He was the 'General' in command.

"So, what are you visualising today?" I asked.

"Prussian soldiers. Frederick the Great's army."

Years later we discovered that Frederick the Great was fondly called, by his people, *Der Alte Fritz.* Why is that relevant? Well, before we discovered that fact, an amazingly loyal, clever, special dog from a rescue centre came into our lives. He was an unwanted black short-haired English collie. And, he came with the name 'Fritz'.

"Why the Prussian army?" I enquired.

"Because they were unbeaten. They were the first to have cavalry ride through the enemy lines and then turn back again. They were armed with just swords, not heavily burdened with all their other equipment." Historian, Robert M. Citino describes Frederick's strategic approach:

> 'In war... he usually saw one path to victory, and that was fixing the enemy army in place, manoeuvring near or even around it to give himself a favourable position for the attack, and then smashing it with an overwhelming blow from an unexpected direction. He was the most aggressive field commander of the century, perhaps of all time, and one who constantly pushed the limits of the possible.'

> Citino, Robert M. *The German Way of War: From the Thirty Years' War to the Third Reich* (University Press of Kansas, 2008), p. 36.

'Pushed the limits of the possible'. Yes, I liked that. Good choice, Steve.

As a child, military history and battle tactics fascinated Steve. I didn't realise that he had remembered so much of it, but I was so glad that he had. Sometimes, I think, we store things away in memory because we know on some level that we're going to need it one day. He continued, "I see the Prussian army riding in and chopping the cancer to bits. Those bits go into my stomach, then to my bowels to be shit out, or to my mouth to be thrown up! Either way, it's out of my body! Like the tides of the sea, relentless – riding back and forth – destroying the cancer enemy for me."

"Why yell 'F'off?'"

"It's my battle charge. The battle cry of the soldiers as they blast through, eliminating it! Oh, and I do it just to annoy you!" he laughed.

What was really happening here? Could Steve's battle visualisation work? Was it, in itself, a form of spiritual healing? He was using the power of imagination, an emotional 'charge' and an unshakeable belief in his own capacity to martial 'forces' that would overwhelm even the most deadly of diseases. Was doing this, every day, actually helping his immune system repair his damaged cells? We believed it was. So, several times a day, he instructed his body's defences – reprogramming the cells of his own body, and I followed Steve's lead – it felt the right thing to do.

Steve saw cavalrymen, but I had an image of battleground nurses like Florence Nightingale, surrounding Steve. Each nurse was ensphered by an aura of golden light. They would reach forward and transfer their light to Steve, flooding his body with a vibrant, pulsating energy. This light strengthened the soldiers and replenished Steve's 'helpful' cells. I felt my visualisation complemented what Steve's was doing, but hopefully with a little less blood and guts flying around.

But, what about the effects of the chemotherapy? Was it doing more harm than good – destroying all the cells – good or bad – in its toxic path? As Dr Kitt said, 'it was lethal stuff'. Was it possibly shortening Steve's precious life; likely to kill him? Or was it just part of the arsenal we needed?

We were keeping to our plan, formed by instinct – surrounding ourselves with only positivity, laughter and life; doing our visualisations daily and being open to all forms of healing, including 'hands-on healing'. All aspects of the plan were carried out with passion, with a stubborn single-mindedness and the powers that be, in this world and beyond, gathered around us.

When the healing sisters, Doreen and Dot, from Wolverhampton Spiritualist Church visited to give Steve 'spiritual healing', I would watch Steve's face and body relax at their touch – a feeling of peacefulness swept over him, one that he was unable to achieve by any other means, as sleep alone could not remove the pain. At night in bed he would be restless, his face troubled, jaw clenched, tossing and turning, moaning in pain and sweat. Yet under the hands of Doreen and Dot he seemed tranquil, calm. It was entrancing to watch, and the sense of peacefulness and love they brought into the room washed over me too. For Steve it was a much-needed respite from the battle zone. 'Reinforcements' for his troops.

When they'd gone he seemed re-energized, more alert, calmer, stronger and even more positive than before. It was like he'd tapped into a source of energy beyond himself – like an infinite, life-giving battery; something from beyond this material world of struggle and confusion.

Doreen told us about The Healing Minute, "Sit by yourselves or with a group at ten o'clock every morning and night and tune into the healing energy. People around the world send healing to those in need at that time. Send your focused healing thoughts and prayers out to those you know who need healing and to those who are asking for help," she told me, "And Steve, open yourself up to receive it."
So I spread the word. Paul, Angie, Sonia, Simon, my dad, Steve and I honoured it every night from then on. We wrote people's names in my healing book so they too could benefit.

"Some people say spiritual healing is all rubbish, but I 'know' something is happening." I ventured to Steve. "Something's going on, but I don't know what," he replied. I felt the tension in my shoulders melt under his words. He knew it too, I was sure.
I postulated to myself 'is healing a greater, higher form of love? Is the thing we call our 'spirit' the means by which we tap into that source of unconditional love? I know we are 'all energy', vibrating away, so if a person is ill or has cancer does it mean that they are vibrating at the incorrect speed or vibration? Can a 'healer' help change that because they are able to vibrate at the right wavelength or vibration? And, by 'resonance' can a healer help bring the patient back into attunement and the correct vibration necessary to regain health?' So many questions to answer.
But, when I asked Steve, "How do you feel after having 'healing'?" he'd just reply, "It's relaxing."

Chapter 15: Too Fragile for Sex!

I looked over at Steve. He was wasting away so swiftly. Most of his hair (from his head and entire body) had abandoned him now; it happened almost overnight, not long after Alex had taken the first fistful in his boisterous game. I recall finding what looked like a black sheepskin rug on the cream bedroom carpet and a dark halo surrounding Steve's head on his pillow. I secreted a lock of his hair in my dressing gown pocket as I silently cleared away the black curls.

What could I do to help him now? I was helpless, just standing by as Steve shrank away before my eyes. I'd heard others call it 'watching the slow death'.

Today Steve announced sadly, "I can't stand. My legs won't hold me."

Shit. Would this be too much for him?

For weeks we had been supporting him to move around from bed to toilet and back again.

I looked at his legs full on for the first time. God he was thin! Skin like tracing paper stretched over protruding bones. He reminded me of the images I'd seen of people starving in concentration camps. So frail, I could imagine his legs snapping under the smallest amount of weight.

Steve and I had always been active – dance classes, martial arts, badminton. He was my six foot 3, well built, athletic partner. We were those youngsters taking jazz ballet classes in the late 70s.

The same images came flooding back to both of us.

"I can't believe you used to wear that bright-blue Lycra leotard and leg warmers. Straight out of 'Fame'," laughed Steve.

"Huh, I remember *you* doing jetty jumps and twirls down the dance studio!" I reminded him. "Imagine being thrown around an Aikido mat now – unbelievable what our bodies went through."

"I am sure we will both get back to it. Anyway, you need to get stronger if you want to be a champion fencer."

This thought prompted me to phone Reg. He would get Steve walking again, I was sure.

Reg, a sports physiotherapist and family friend, was such a passionate, positive man. I had asked him to visit Steve just after he was first diagnosed in hospital – as he too had fought the battle with cancer and won. Reg believed it was mind over matter In fact, he had refused treatment and discharged himself from the hospital. Drastic I thought, but… he was alive and well still – five years later.

Steve laughed when he told me about Reg's parting words to him, "He said if I didn't get off my arse and beat this, he would kick my sorry ass around the ward until I did!"

Reg was one of his heroes. He believed that what seemed impossible could actually be achieved, and knew ways to dismantle the barriers that held people back. As the physiotherapist for Britain's entry to the World's Strongest Man competition, he had supported athletes working at the outer limits of physical endurance and – closer to home – had worked on me for many years since my first ice skating injury. He had spurred me on when I was in so much pain that I wanted to give in. He had an unusual approach, but it worked. I can still remember him making me laugh with rallying calls such as, "Come on Mandy, get your tits off the bed!" as I struggled to do the exercises he prescribed.

My poor spine suffered from the damage caused by the many skating falls and the pressure I put on myself to perform beyond my own physical boundaries. I did not want to give up doing my sports. Reg showed me how to protect myself, how to strengthen my spine and give it the rest it needed to recover from the abuse it took. But more than this, he told me so many inspiring stories. I have always loved to hear how people find their way through hardship and realise their will to succeed, in whatever way that might be. We can all learn from each other.

One I remember was of a young girl who had become paraplegic as a result of a traffic accident and just lay in bed giving up on her life. Her parents called Reg in to help. He identified the few muscles that she could use to get her sitting and, having regained some of her physical confidence, Reg got her swimming and even winning competitions.

Steve and my dad first met Reg at the Corinthian Gym in Wolverhampton. Reg had been there supporting my dad in his training in the lead up to his world sit-up record attempt. Dad had wanted to do something to raise money for deaf children. He had always boasted about his strong stomach muscles, so sit-ups seemed the way to go. However, not sit-ups from the flat surface of the floor; that would be too easy. My dad did them on an inclined bench, making it even harder! At the age of 52, Dad managed 2000 sit-ups in 44 minutes, all witnessed by the Guinness World Record officials and the local press. If anyone could motivate Steve to do the impossible it was Reg; he would know how to help him, I was certain.

Reg got down to business with his usual no-nonsense approach.
"Right, this is the plan of action. Mandy, I'll teach you how to massage Steve's legs. You will have to do it every day, just as I show you. It is vital we keep the muscles in his legs stimulated, so the blood continues to flow to them. And, exercises are important too. Until he can move his legs himself you will need to do the exercises for him, by moving his legs." He then pointed to Steve, "You will help as much as possible, no laziness!"
So began my lessons and our new daily regime. Could I do it though?

I was scared to touch Steve in case I hurt him. To me, he was egg-shell fragile. He was in constant pain. Even lying next to him as I slept was a worry. So how could I yank his legs about, carrying out these strenuous physical exercises? But, Reg taught me techniques that visibly relaxed Steve, and I could feel his muscles soften under my hands. I realised that he was teaching me something highly valuable. It was a healing art that I

87

found myself wanting to practise more. I felt called to develop it and later went on to qualify in Swedish massage and aromatherapy. These weren't the same techniques, though, that Reg taught me. I believe he said that he had learned them from a Korean source.

We managed to maintain some strength and movement in Steve's body, by religiously carrying out these exercises. Steve didn't complain (much), though I'm sure it was uncomfortable at times. Nonetheless, as time progressed we both made a decision. It wasn't a spoken decision, but a natural one. His frail body could not find the strength for us to sustain the physical sexual connection, which we loved so much. Steve could not take my weight, or his own. He became too weak and in too much pain. He was simply too fragile for sex. Sex is such a major part of most young couples' lives. It certainly was for us. Looking back, though, I realise that the intimacy of touch became our new sex life. We grew closer through touch, even more connected. Just holding hands can be so important. I love to see elderly couples, walking, hand in hand. It's an expression of intimacy and trust, connection and love. I always had a surge of happiness when I saw my own parents and grandparents hold hands. It's a sacred, special connection that should not be reserved for teenagers!

Chapter 16: Another Nail in the Coffin

One morning a brown envelope dropped on the doormat. I could tell immediately that it was from the Benefits Agency. Good – Sandra had said we would definitely get help given our circumstances. Now I'd be able to put Steve's mind at rest. I knew it wouldn't be a lot, not as much as Steve earned, but at least it would keep the mortgage secure and give us some money for food and other bills. One headache less. The sick pay had ceased from Crown Paints last month, but they were kind enough to let us keep the car for the time being. They sent me a gift too!

A bouquet of lilies, gerbera daisies, roses and sunflowers arrived one morning. What a surprise! To me a bouquet of flowers heralds celebration or thanks. Less than a year ago, after coming home with our new baby, Alex, Steve had given me a bounteous armful of flowers to mark the wonderful arrival of our son. So, I suppose I did have mixed feelings about the Crown Paints bouquet.

Interflora delivered them. The card read 'To Mandy, thinking of you, Crown Paints'. I pondered the message on the flower card. Who had supplied the wording? Why 'Crown Paints' and not the names of the colleagues he'd worked with?

No doubt they had agonised over it. What would I have written? 'Our prayers are with you'? But, wasn't that what you write when someone has just died? What about 'Best Wishes'? No, too lame, an understatement – I might say that to an elderly aunt on her birthday.

'Thought this might cheer you up' – too trivial in the circumstances, as if to imply you've no right to be sad anyway. Yes, a difficult task, but the bouquet was a wonderful surprise. It did make me spontaneously smile that day. I love receiving flowers. Those flowers made me feel thought of – someone out there knew I was going through really difficult times and wanted to let me know that they felt for me. It's that simple really. The words on the card were unimportant in a way. I understood what was intended.

I trailed my hands through the Crown Paint flowers as I passed the vase. Only a few life-clutching blooms remained in their full splendour. I wanted them to last forever. A reminder to me of the kindness of others.

"Steve! Good news," I shouted up the stairs. "We've had a letter from the Benefits Agency." I started to open it, as I climbed the stairs. I was eager to see what we'd been given, but as I unfolded the paper, the words that caught my eye utterly astounded me. I stood speechless for a spilt second. I thought 'first the cashing in of the insurance policy and now this!' It caught me off guard and for a moment my positive determination wavered. This was a cruel joke.

"What's it say?" Steve's voice penetrated my stupor. I looked at him. "You are not going to believe this one. 'They' obviously know something we don't." I sat down on the bed, shaking my head. I suppose I should have cried, but instead I laughed. I just *had* to laugh at this. I had no choice. "I've been awarded my Widow's Pension!"

"What? Bloody cheek! I'm not dead yet!"

I had been expecting Income Support, Attendance Allowance or something similar to see us through, but not this. I looked again at the offending (hopefully not prophetic) letter, my hands shaking. Yes, it was addressed to me and yes I had scanned it correctly. I, Mandy Brown, in the eyes of the government was already a 'Widow'. I looked at Steve, my apparently 'deceased' husband.

We both said the exact same thing at the exact same time, "I can't believe this!" which simultaneously made us both laugh too.

Calmly I picked up the phone and dialled the number at the top of the letter. I explained, some levity in my voice, to the unsuspecting soul at the end of the line, "You have sent me my Widow's Pension."

Expectant, "Yes?"

With barely suppressed indignation in my voice, tempered with just a little black humour, I continued, "Problem is, just two minutes ago, when I last checked, my husband – he was still alive. He may well be terribly ill with cancer, but he is not quite dead yet!"

Silence.

"Yes, he is terminally ill – I will give you that – but he is still just about breathing, he has a pulse, he's hanging on in there." I took a deep breath. "Look, I know you personally might not have made this mistake, but I am NOT a widow, not yet at least, and I hope I don't become one soon either!"

To this day I cannot understand how they managed to make that cruel mistake. I recall the mortified woman at the end of the phone mumbling and stuttering her apologies on behalf of Work and Pensions. We got our Income Support (the benefit we were expecting) remarkably quickly thereafter.

In a way the whole episode was laughable really – Steve and I had a giggle about it as we pictured the embarrassed faces, listening to my rant. But in the quiet moments later on, my mind kept returning to that letter – was it an omen; did it reflect what was the inevitable future for us both? Was the universe giving me a reality check? God, I hoped not. I pushed the ugly thought away. It was just a simple mistake, a computer glitch... wasn't it?

Chapter 17: Midnight call

The early hours of the morning were a peaceful, serene time of contemplation for me. I gazed at Steve's restless form beside me. He was wasting away – becoming more insubstantial each day. I gently stroked his palm, which I knew soothed him like a lullaby.

I jumped at the shrill sound of the phone ringing. 'Argh, don't wake him' my mind screamed as I lashed out for the receiver.

"Mandy, it's Grant. I used to work with Steve. I've just heard, and I needed to ring you tell you he will be okay." Grant? Who was Grant? I didn't recognise the voice and I couldn't place him among the people Steve used to talk about from work. It was past midnight but he obviously thought his call important. I allowed him to continue.

"Steve will be okay" he insisted, "You see, I died and came back."

I sat upright in bed.

"What?"

"I died and I need to tell you what happened. It will help Steve."

Years later I penned this letter, but did not have a full name or address to which to send it:

Dear Grant,
I apologize as I can't really remember speaking you be-
fore or after that call, but I want you to know that you
did make a real impact that night. Thank you for having
the courage to phone me – a stranger – and share your

story. It truly did help. I hope you are still fit and well today wherever you are. I believe you will be out there somewhere enjoying life to the full. I have told your story many times over the years to help others in pain and fear of death – so thank you our friend – you made a difference!
Much love
Mandy & Steve

Grant explained,
"The first thing I remember was looking at someone in a bed and thinking 'God he's in a bad way, poor bugger'. I didn't recognize the place. I could hear voices so I went to investigate. My vision seemed off, wider somehow. In the next room, I saw a woman behind a desk – a nurse judging by the uniform – with an array of grey and red pigeon holes set in the wall behind her. She was talking on the phone. I was just about to attract her attention when alarms sounded and bright flashing lights interrupted us. Suddenly people – nurses and doctors – appeared from nowhere, rushing into the room I'd just been in. It was loud, frantic, confusing: voices shouting instructions, machines beeping and bleeping, syringes being filled. But, no one seemed to notice me as they hooked up the resuscitation machine to that guy. Each time one of them shouted, 'All clear!' his body leaped up above the bed by several inches and danced violently in the air. *I* thought the guy looked 'well dead' already to be honest.

"We've lost him! He's gone," the doctor decided.

I remember the doctor was short with dark scruffy hair and corduroy trousers.

The same doctor asked, "Time of death, nurse?"

I moved in to take a closer look. I wanted to see the face of the man they'd tried in vain to save. It didn't feel wrong for me to get nearer. I knew I had some connection to him. I gazed down on him and took note of the familiar features; the face of someone I knew so well. It was me, Mandy. *I* was the dead guy in the bed.

I was in intensive care. I'd been on my motorbike, was hit by a car and now... I had died. I was outside of my body, but still fully aware, conscious, and able to think. I could hear the conversations – catching the names of those still around my bed: Dr Graham, Nurse Stokes, John. I felt free and peaceful, just observing the situation from a detached point of view. I had so many questions, like how am I going to tell my parents? Why hadn't I noticed earlier that I was seeing the whole scene from above? How come I now had what seemed like 180-degree vision? Can I control this floating body? Indeed, when I thought of the nurses' station, I appeared back there staring at the pigeon holes again.

But then my vision blurred. I felt a strong pulling sensation, as if I'd been grabbed from behind and slammed onto the floor. The force of it was unbelievably strong, like being hit by a train. And the pain, oh my God, it was so intense! But I knew I was back in my body and I did not like it. I blacked out.

When I awoke my dad was sitting at my bedside. I was
eager to talk about what happened as I could recall being 'dead', yet no one – my dad, the nurse – no one
mentioned it at that time. The drugs made me drowsy
and I was in and out of consciousness, for about a week
or so, I'm told. When conscious I desperately wanted to
get back out of my body to escape the pain which
flooded through me.

You must tell Steve. Is he in pain?"
"Yes."
"When I was out of my body, when I died, I was free of
pain even when they tried to resuscitate me. I realised
that now I was back in my body, so to speak, there
might be a way to get out of my body again – as a
means of escape. If I could get out of my body – even
partially or temporarily – I would be free of the unbearable pain. It works, believe me.
Tell Steve to imagine he is rocking, but not to move
physically. Rock himself out of his body and hover just
a few centimetres above it. That's what I did and I managed to perfect this technique, and to gain hours of relief several times a day. I did it for months when I was
convalescing in the hospital.
We survive after death. I am one hundred per cent sure
of it and we can get out of our bodies!"

"So Grant, did anyone confirm you'd died?"
"I asked my dad. He was amazed that I knew. I asked
him if I'd been brought in via the nurses' station and he
said no, I came in through the other emergency door
from theatre. So I couldn't know about the grey and red

pigeon holes unless I had been there in 'spirit', so to speak."

"I do believe we are spirits in a body, Grant." I said. "Dr Graham confirmed it: I had died for several minutes, failed to be resuscitated, he started to pronounce me dead, but then they tried one more time to shock me back and it worked. Nurse Stokes was the one sitting at reception."

"Thanks, Grant. I will tell Steve."

Grant's story reminded me of a certain conversation I had had with my dad in the café at the ice rink when I was a teenager. I can recall the scene clearly...

"It amazes me how you can balance a tray of full tea cups and walk in your skates so gracefully," Dad said. I looked around to see others wobbling in their bright-blue skates as they staggered over the rubber floor trying not to spill their single coffee cup.

"Practice!" I said.

What prompted the topic I brought up next I will never know but, out of the blue, I asked my dad, "What do you think happens when we die?"

"Nothing. We just rot in the earth," he replied matter-of-factly.

"No, I mean to *us*, not our bodies."

"Nothing happens."

"After we die, when *we* continue – our spirit I mean. What happens to our spirit?"

Dad looked at me blankly.

I realised that day that he did not know something that I *knew* so clearly, so deeply, without any doubt – he did not know we survived after the death of our bodies.

97

"Your consciousness, the thinking part of you – what happens to that? What happens to the real you, the real Charlie?"

"I don't know."

I was astonished. He meant it.

I looked at him as if seeing him for the first time. His eyes met mine and I, fleetingly, felt he was surprised that *I* could be his lifeline.

I felt sorry for him, and concerned for him, "Dad, I have always known our spirit, our soul or our consciousness – whatever you want to call it – continues in some form after the body dies. I just know it's true!" I could not believe my dad did not. I thought we all knew our spirit survived, and people just disagreed as to where it goes.

Chapter 18: Deadliner

"Tomorrow I will feel better!" was Steve's daily mantra as he prepared to attempt another night's sleep. They were the last words I heard, muttered quietly under his breath, as I drifted into my own fitful sleep. I wanted to stay awake for Steve, be there for him until he was asleep, but invariably exhaustion took over. I knew that he hardly slept at all these days. The pain was too intense and even the morphine was having little effect. I would often wake up and look across at him, seeing him, eyes open, and know immediately that he had experienced yet another torturous night without the respite of sleep. What did he think of during those deathly, quiet hours?

I joined him in his waking vigil the night before his next review appointment. It had been six-and-a-half months since his terminal diagnosis. Yes, over six months! I tried to hold onto the fact that Steve was very much *still* alive and breathing. Mr Rogers had been wrong – Steve had survived well beyond his allotted three months, so we just had to keep going. Surely the cancer would give up before Steve did!

"How do you feel today?" I probed.
"Fine, fine."
"No seriously, tell me the truth."
"Well, I have had three doses of poison so far and lots of healing from Doreen. I feel okay, pain's a bugger still, but I'm not giving up."

Yes, Steve was definitely more positive in himself – brighter in some ways. Maybe the 'spiritual' healing and all those prayers were helping. I bloody hoped so. Only Mr Rogers, my dad, Steve's parents and I were privy to the 'three month sell by date/death sentence' itself. I had insisted that no one else was told – after all how could Mr Rogers be sure; he was not a God.

Dr Kitt ushered us into the examination room with a brief smile. Dr K (as we now called him) was starting to grow on me. He did not say much; you could say he lacked warmth but I felt sure he was the right oncologist for us – thorough, persistent and determined to keep his patients alive.

He prodded and probed Steve's stomach. We waited in a hushed silence.
"Mmm."
"How am I doing?" Steve was eager to know.
"Mmm, not good." His face looked grave.
"Oh." Steve simply replied.

Dr K shook his head and looked up at me. The ticking of the clock in the room hammered in my head. I desperately wanted – needed – Dr K to tell me it was going to be okay. In my mind I was begging him to say, 'Steve is healing. The cancer is shrinking. He is going to live'.
"No, the chemotherapy is not working. The tumours have grown. I cannot feel any organs due to the size of the tumours. Steve, you must be in a lot of pain. I will increase the morphine dose to help."

Steve numbly nodded his head but did not speak.

'No, no, no!' the voice in my head screamed as my eyes betrayed me, oozing tears. No, I must hold back, no sobbing, I must be strong. I'd promised myself, Steve and all the powers that be. The recollection of this somehow helped me focus. Steve stared at the ceiling. I could just feel his devastation. It felt like his will to fight, his life force was draining out of him. I squeezed his hand. No response.

Dr K started tidying away, closing Steve's folder. No, it cannot end like this.

"But," I blurted out, not sure what to say next. I just had to re-engage Dr K, "Dr Kitt you have to do something. Steve has felt so much better lately. We were sure he was beating it. That he was getting better."

To my pleading expression he replied, "Sorry. The chemotherapy has not had the effect I wanted."

'Stop saying that!' my inner voice yelled. I looked at Steve – still no reaction. 'Please don't give up my love, please don't.' That bloody clock ticked away, even louder, threatening to overwhelm me. I had to fight for Steve. I had to find the words he could not.

"So what are you going to try next? You said you would keep trying different types of chemo until... well, if one did not work you mentioned that there were lots of chemo drugs and combinations you could try. Will you?"

He looked at me quizzically. He must have felt the force of my will, coming straight at him across that consulting room – it was tangible to me – I was projecting 'don't you dare say 'no'!' Steve stirred, seeming to regain awareness of what was going on. He turned to look at Dr K for his answer.

We were greeted with silence. There was no emotion on Dr K's face; nothing to give away what he was thinking, how he would respond. So we waited.

He opened up his notes again, looked at them, pulled out the x-rays once more and started to scribble something down on a piece of paper. With an inscrutable face he handed it to Steve.

"Come in next week for some more blood tests. You need to get your blood count up."

"And if they are up?" I asked, fearful that the consultation was over and he would offer no more hope.

"We'll see," and he left the room.

'We'll see' – what did that mean? I knew it would be unhelpful to continue badgering Dr K, to call him back. I just had to try to turn that 'we'll see' statement into a more positive statement. Steve silently and slowly got dressed.

As we drove home my mind worked overtime, frantically searching for signs, clues, hints of Steve's continued survival. Meanwhile next to me I could feel his faith in our plan – his mission to remain alive – diminishing. He was slipping away from me and I didn't know how to stop it. He was unusually quiet. I could

only hope he too was searching for reasons to continue
believing, to keep trying.

He needed time alone. I needed to give him that time,
but I can tell you I was scared. What if he gave up now?
It was that three months curse. Mr Rogers was right.
Steve had been lucky to have that extra three months. It
was a postponement, but not a reprieve. I was stupid,
selfish, living an illusion.

As soon as we got home, Steve went upstairs to bed. I
sat downstairs and quietly cried; forcing myself to hold
in the sobs that shook my body. Alex came up to me.
He gently climbed up onto my lap and curled his little
arms around me, holding me, giving me comfort when I
needed it most. My silent tears dropped onto his head,
but he never stirred or moved. Bless him. He knew
something was wrong. My little Alexander was my
rock of strength. Thank you, Alex.

Chapter 19: Dying for Cold Turkey

Drowning, I felt like I was drowning. Panic and fear gripped me. Like a giant octopus grabbing and pulling me beneath the waves to the depths of despair – its tentacles wrapping around me with its sole intent to immobilise me, squeezing out all hope and life. I felt unable to move, to escape, to fight.

I heard a voice from somewhere scream, "Get help!"

I pushed it away. It was too late. Steve was dying. I couldn't stop it. I thought I could – if I kept positive enough, strong enough, believed enough. But I'd failed. 'I am so sorry Steve,' I moaned.

Dr K and Mr Rodgers were in agreement. Time was up. Nothing left to be done. It was so unfair. He was, we were too young. What about Alex? He needed a father. I needed a lover, a husband, a soul mate. I wouldn't cope without him. I just knew it. Had I wasted those three months chasing an illusion, an unrealisable dream, built on my own selfish desires? I felt racked with guilt and such a deep, deep pain of aching, all-encompassing sadness. The demon of self-pity had arrived again.

I sat bolt upright, in defiance. NO! There must be something more I could do. I was not going to give up the fight.

I pushed away the creeping darkness and probed my memory, my imagination, my logical mind, my spirit for ideas. Steve was so weak. It was up to me to help him – to 'get help'. What could I do now? Whose help could I ask for? Then it came to me – Doreen! I needed Doreen to help me bring Steve back from the precipice.

She wouldn't give up on him, even if all the doctors in the world had – I felt sure of it.

Doreen came around immediately after my phone call. Steve remained upstairs in bed, immersed in his own growing despair.
She turned to me first of all. "Let's give *you* some healing," she said.
"What about Steve?"
"You need it more at the moment. Anyway, I have a book for Steve to read, if he wants to."
Unsure I took the book up to Steve. Well at least it might take his mind off things – if he would read it. Steve wasn't a big reader.
I left Steve flicking though it. The book was about a healer called Harry Edwards. That was all I knew.

I couldn't help but feel a little guilty when Doreen sat me down, and told me to close my eyes.
"Just accept the healing. It will make you stronger. Steve is fine for a few minutes. You need to relax and recharge."
True. So I allowed myself to just sit awhile and regroup my thoughts. As the moments passed I felt an oozing of warmth spread from Doreen's fingers into my tense shoulder muscles. Sighing in relaxation, I felt a loving energy encompass me, hold me and soothe me. Bliss. I did not understand how this healing thing worked but it was so calming and peaceful. Soft tears fell down my cheek. They were not tears of sadness though, but of release, of joy or contentment even. I felt protected and

loved. I felt as if everything would be all right. I wanted to stay in that safe, loving atmosphere.

The healing session was over too soon. Doreen hugged me, saying "God Bless." Floating on a cloud of serenity, I smiled my gratitude. The air around us seemed to vibrate with a feeling of harmony and love. I know it sounds silly, but that is how it felt.

The peace, however, was shattered seconds later by a shout from Steve,

"Right that's it! Fucked if they think they're going to kill me off! Mandy! Mandy!"

As I raced upstairs, Doreen nodded and walked into the kitchen saying, "I'll make the tea and bring it up."

Steve thrust the book at me, "Look at this!"

He seemed half way through it already, I noticed.

"It says here that when the doctors are preparing people to die they up the morphine dose. I am way above the recommended morphine dose for 'dying patients'. Bloody morphine doesn't work anyway – makes me feel shit and I am still in agony!"

At that moment I knew Steve was ready to fight on.

He announced, "Right that's it. I am going to stop all the morphine – it's not helping me. I'd rather be in pain and think straight, than on morphine and doped up to the eyeballs!"

Wow, that was exactly what I wanted to hear, but… reason kicked in soon after,

"Steve you can't just stop it overnight. You have to come off slowly. You have been taking morphine for nearly a year now."
"Don't care. It stops now!"

Steve wanted to take back control of his body, so he could reclaim his life. This much I understood. But I feared the pain would increase beyond endurance. I did not want him to suffer excruciating pain. As if he heard my thoughts, he said,
"I already *am* in excruciating pain. It can't get any worse!"

And stop he did – that same day. This is when the 'fun' started!

Echoing through the house were cries of, "Mandy get the maggots off my legs!"
I detest and abhor those loathsome creatures. Steve used to take maggots fishing and I couldn't bear to look at them. To even contemplate that some fishermen put them in their mouths – urghh! Yes, I know they are part of nature's great web of life and that hospitals have been known to use them to treat open infections, but really... the mere thought of hundreds of maggots all squirming and wriggling over each other was enough to make me hurl! I shudder at the slightest glimpse.

"Mandy, quick brush them off!" Of all the nightmare images Steve's subconscious might contain, I couldn't believe it was maggots that he dredged up for his hallucination! He was convinced that his itching legs were

107

covered with those hideous wrigglers. I knew there were none there but dutifully I wiped them away for him, knowing it would comfort him. Meanwhile I tried not to allow my imagination to fill in the blank space. I loved Steve but honestly, at this moment, I wished our thoughts were not always so in tune.

Steve was experiencing 'cold turkey'. Withdrawal from opiates comes at a high price. He seemed to be sweating one minute and shivering with cold the next. His hallucinations came and went and came again for weeks. He was fixated with his legs, always trying to shake off the imagined maggots!

True to his word, and as a testament to his strength of character, my Steve never had another morphine tablet or injection from that day onwards. What would Dr K say to that?

Chapter 20: Feel the Fear and Do it Anyway

Steve was off the morphine and I felt that we had made a step forward of a different kind. It was strange territory but we were going to plough ahead. He seemed brighter these days. His spirits had lifted. Perhaps overcoming the morphine withdrawal had proven something to him about the art of the possible. But he still took me by surprise when he quietly asked me that question, "How do I pray?"

"What?" I was shocked. I knew it had been difficult for him to ask that question, because behind it lay a whole avalanche of mental turmoil; of considering the prospect of his own death and what might happen after death, of questioning if there was a higher power in the universe that might help us and can that power be called upon to help fight against our own mortality, to conquer death (if only for a time)?

"I don't really know."

"Other people pray. They pray for me. You pray too I think."

I nodded, yes I suppose I did pray in my own way.

"What do you do? I think I should pray."

Steve waited patiently for me to formulate an answer.

"I don't know. I just say my thoughts in my head and hope someone is listening… "

Not a great answer.

"I think we should talk about me dying. I've been thinking. I want you to take some photographs of me as I am now. Just in case I die. I want Alex to have some photographs of him with his dad."

I sat Alex on the bed with Steve and they both dutifully posed for the camera. "Please," I silently prayed, "don't let this be the last photo I have of Steve." I promised myself that as soon as Steve looked better I would take another photo of them together.

Yet as I looked through Alex's first year of baby photos later that night, I had to admit Steve looked increasingly worse, fading away with such pain in his eyes, as that year progressed. I couldn't bear to look at the evidence, so I hid the book away.

Steve sat up in bed and attempted to pray properly for the first time. He had not slept for such a long time. He really needed some rest.

"Please, oh please help him," my thoughts begged, silently supporting him in my own prayers. "If only he could sleep, I am sure he would feel better, be stronger."

An image of Doreen came into my mind. She believed anyone could heal. That mothers did it naturally in response to their children's cries or illnesses. All she did differently was ask to be used as a channel for that healing energy.

"Please use me for healing," I silently implored, "Please let the healing energy flow through me to Steve. Help him please."

'Oh shit, oh no… This can't be happening, not again'. I remembered this feeling, from so long ago. Anxiety swept over me as I was transported back to my childhood.

It started when I was around six years old. Lying in bed I had felt the slow progression. It always started with my fingers. A numbing, tingly sensation that made me stare at my fingers as if they were going to transform into something else. It was as if they were growing, swelling, puffing out. They still looked like *my* fingers and hands, but they felt huge.

Sometimes it stopped there – at that 'big hands' stage. Other times it progressed further, into what I called the 'super-sensitive' stage. I could feel every little imperfection in my fingers. I would frantically try to find something smooth to touch. I'd reach out for the melamine surface of my bedroom dresser thinking it was super smooth – no, it has tiny scratches and bumps. I'd reach for the polished wooden bed frame – no full of ridges, so slight I would never normally notice. Everything I touched had minute marks, a subtle but unmistakeable texture I could only feel when this happened to my hands. This super-sensitivity touch would then pass to my mouth. I could feel, with my tongue, every microscopic imperfection in the enamel surface of my teeth – not pleasant. But you know what? At least it encouraged me to keep my teeth regularly brushed!

I asked my mum about it.
"What is it? Does it happen to you? Why does it happen?"
She didn't know and, I suppose to protect me, she passed it off as me being silly or having 'nerves'. Whatever it was, I felt my mother was a little scared of it. Consequently, I grew up being scared of it too.

111

And now here I was, an adult, experiencing that same weird sensation again: the huge hands, the super-sensitivity. It was like being in a supernatural, horror movie having some paranormal powers conferred on me and having no idea where they came from or how to control it. Of course, I panicked.

I don't know how long it took, but eventually I scolded myself. 'Hold on, hold on… this can't be a bad thing. You have just asked for help. To be used for healing. To help Steve. This can't be a bad thing or just a coincidence.' Without any further thought or doubt I gently placed my hands on Steve's side. He stirred and half opened his eyes.

"Mmm, that's nice. Where did you get the hot water bottle from?"

"Steve look," I could barely breathe out the words, "it's not a hot water bottle, it's my hands!"

"Bloody hell!" was his reply.

I chuckled and, keeping my hands on him, I explained, "I asked to be used for healing, like Doreen said, and well… my hands have… changed, gone hot."

"Well, just keep them there. Your hands are usually freezing – makes a nice change!" I couldn't agree more. So I kept my hands in place and continued to ask for healing for Steve… if only to give him a night's rest.

Amazingly, within a short while, Steve drifted off to sleep. I didn't dare move for fear of waking him. I admit – I felt pleased with myself.

When he was still sound asleep a few hours later, my hands still touching his sides, I did gently pull back. What had happened? I just kept looking at Steve and wondering what this all meant.

The following morning on stirring from sleep, sheer dread hit me. Steve lay motionless beside me. He was always awake when I woke up, but not today. I reached out my hand to check the temperature of his body. He was cold. Fear rose from the pit of my stomach. What had I done? I'd asked to help him sleep. I didn't mean forever. Irrationality surfed the bed covers like a tidal wave. My mind raced. Had I killed him? Put him out of his misery – put him 'to sleep'? I didn't want this! Oh my God, what had I done?

"Morning," his voice rose up from the sheets, groggy but certainly alive. I felt the weight lift from my chest – and air flowed into my lungs again. For a few awful seconds – that had seemed like long hours – I had lived through his death and it had nearly crushed me. But he was still alive!

Before he even saw my face, I could hear the panic and concern in his voice, "What's wrong? Are you okay?" This was so typical of Steve, such an indication of our deep connection, that whenever I was upset or in pain, some psychic alarm went off inside him. He automatically put me first – before his own pains and concerns. He was constantly concerned for me, even though he was the one that was so poorly.

"I thought I'd killed you. When I woke up you were so still."

"Oh!" he nodded now realising what I meant. "Yes, I must have dropped off. Amazing. What happened?"

"Dropped off? Excuse the pun, but you slept like the dead! I watched you for hours. I was so pleased you were finally sleeping that I was scared to go to sleep… in case you didn't wake up. And when I did wake up you were so still, and so cold to the touch, I thought I *had* killed you."

"Can't get rid of me that easily!" Steve pulled me to him and I nestled in his embrace.

Doreen knowingly smiled when we told our strange story. I had an uncanny feeling that this would not be the last we heard of it either.

Chapter 21 : Crypt Humour

"Dr K's secretary just rang. Your blood count's up again." Relief surged through me, "He has agreed, you can start chemo again on Friday!"

"Great" said Steve with mock excitement, "That will be as much fun as pulling toenails. Can't wait!"

So back to the Crypt he returned. Dr K warned, "Steve, your attitude to fighting this is the only reason I have agreed to keep treating you, but I believe it is just prolonging the inevitable."

***

It was visiting time. I would recognise Steve's laughter anywhere. Hearing it as soon as I came onto the ward always made me smile, but as I turned the corner and caught sight of him, my stomach clenched. He looked so frail. His skin – tissue-paper thin. 'Breathe deep and smile' I told myself.

"Hiya, Steve," I leaned over to kiss him, aware once again, of that odd smell like rotting flesh coming from his body. 'Hospital smell' I told myself, firmly, 'from the chemotherapy'. I shook my head to dispel the niggling alternative. "So what's been happening?"

"That guy, over there, can't get out of bed. He doesn't talk either." Steve pointed to a frail white-haired man in the bed opposite.

"The guy with pensioner blond hair?" I echoed my dad's joke about his own grey hair.

Steve nodded. "The poor bugger keeps shitting the bed. Yesterday we had a laugh though. Mike was put in the bed next to him."

I went to wave to Mike, but he was curled up under his sheets. He and Steve were the same age and their chemo sessions often coincided.

Steve continued, "In the night the old guy must have had a temperature because the nurses got a fan out and put it on his side table." Steve shook his head with a smile, "In the morning I woke up to see Mike retching and heaving."

'Nothing new there' I thought.

Steve put his hand up to attract my attention, "But, get this… Mike was cursing and swearing in between retches. His mum had brought him in some grapes. Mike decided he fancied them that morning. Only when he was eating them, he discovered they had bits of poo on them!"

"Really?"

"The old guy had pooed, kicked off his sheets and the fan blowing in Mike's direction did the rest. No one's fault, but you've gotta laugh!"

"Or throw up!" I replied. A reoccurring thought passed through my head… Steve had the knack of seeing the funny side of life – so encouraging that ability to keep laughing might be another key element in our plan.

Even prior to Steve's illness, our friends would often comment, "You two laugh so much. You are always laughing." And yes, we both saw the funny side of things in life and Steve's humour had got him into trouble many times.

Years later, I would do some research into laughter and find a US author, Norman Cousins, boasting that reruns of Candid Camera and Marx Brothers movies helped him overcome his cancer in the 1970s; Bill Trent reporting that an Ottawa cancer lodge had added 'humour to its armamentarium in the fight against cancer,' and in the NCBI's National Library of Medicine I'd find various studies, including one which stated,

'Laughter may reduce stress and improve NK cell activity. As low NK cell activity is linked to decreased disease resistance and increased morbidity in persons with cancer and HIV disease, laughter may be a useful cognitive-behavioural intervention.'

There were so many opportunities to find the black, humorous side of life on the cancer ward. Bets could be placed on the most unlikely of sports. Like the day when Steve and his Crypt companion, Jim, watched another patient walk slowly up the ward. What marked this poor guy out was the fact that he could not control his flatulence.

"I bet you ten to one," Jim challenged Steve, "that 'Farting Man' (and indeed the man was farting with every step he took) shits himself before he gets to the end of the ward!" Who knows whether he won his bet. I didn't ask.

Dark humour was part of the furniture. Steve asserted that, "Life is not worth living if you can't have a laugh! People take themselves too seriously – they should lighten up a bit."

117

I conceded he may have a point, but often cringed, at the more extreme examples.

"So, what were you just laughing at when I came in?" I asked.

He lay back on his pillow. I could tell he was composing himself to tell me another story.

"Okay, I had two doctors come in yesterday. They decided they wanted to shove cameras up my backside again. 'This is getting a habit,' I said. One doctor asked me, 'Oh can a student come in on this please?' I said 'Yes.'"

I wondered why they wanted to do this procedure. I would ask the nurse later.

"So I turn over, knees up, curtains drawn. I heard shuffling and noise behind me and thought, 'Come on get on with it!' Up goes the bicycle pump tube and up goes a probe.

I turned round and bloody hell…" He paused for effect, "Twelve people all staring at my bare arse! 'What's this – a party?' I asked, 'You said *a* student!'" He mimicked the doctor's response, "'Well as they were all here we thought they may as well.'" Steve huffed, but I knew he did not mind really.

"I have told them I will be selling tickets next week!" I chuckled.

Steve continued, "Gareth – guy in the bed over there – great bloke, you'd like him – he has expressed to me a real concern that they have been up his arse so many times, he thinks that secretly… they are building a ship in a bottle up there!"

"That's brilliant," I laughed.

Steve said, "I said to him… more like a 'shit in a bottle!'"

One of the nurses came to check Steve's drip, "Tell her about the challenge you and Mike have started," she said.

"Oh, yeah. When a nurse comes in, we ask their name… and we have to sing a well-known song containing their name. I am so winning this!"

That did not surprise me. "Examples?" I asked.

"Carol… *Oh, Carol*, Neil Sedaka. Jane… *Baby Jane*, Rod Stewart. Diana? *Diana*, Paul Anka. Maria… easy – *Maria*, West Side Story. We were stumped this afternoon though… Alison?"

Alison? Alison? I couldn't think of one, but then again I can never remember titles or song lyrics.

Steve continued, "After a couple of minutes both Mike and I sang, doing our best Elvis Costello cover… '*AAAAAlison. I know this world is killing you…*'"

I recall there being a real camaraderie in that ward. It was as if they were all conspiring together to beat the gloom; almost everyone pitched in with the jokes and general silliness of the place. Was that usual or was it down to Steve's boisterous influence? I know he's my husband, but I do believe he has a gift for raising the spirits of others. He helped to open people up, get them talking. He would 'talk to anyone' (I so admired his ability to do that) and always made friends. Sharing a ward with Steve was never boring, I felt sure. Even the nurses seemed to join in the fun. He was well liked. Maybe this is why, when he started to be really ill, they

119

too found it difficult to keep smiling and be positive around him.

Chapter 22: Skin the Fish

It always seemed such a solemn occasion collecting
Steve from the Crypt (otherwise known as the Deansley
ward). Dropping him off there was just as bad though.
It was getting more difficult each time. Steve would
complain,
"As soon as I walk up to the door of Deansley ward my
stomach turns, I feel nauseous and start to shiver. I hate
everything it stands for."
I squeezed his bony hand.
Steve continued, "I can smell the chemo drugs down
the corridor, and once I am through the doors the outside world disappears and all focus is on filling my
veins with that bloody poison, until I'm let out of the
'Crypt' again."
I winced in guilt.

Helplessness, that pathetic, feeble creature, always met
me at that exact same door. *She* spun her cobweb of
loneliness around my heart as he looked into my eyes
and kissed me goodbye. As I returned home alone she
sang her melancholic laments in my head. In the last
seven years, Steve and I had spent all our free time together; enjoyed the same sports, hobbies and social life.
My dad even joked once that we were so entwined,
never leaving each other's side, that we were stuck together like 'shit to a blanket'. I didn't like the word
'shit' but I appreciated the meaning.
I remember with pride what happened, a few years
back, when Steve attended an all-male sales training
seminar. The trainer asked everyone how much time,

121

percentage wise, they listened to their friends, work colleagues and their wives or girlfriends. Most of the sales reps gave low numbers when it came to wives and girlfriends, but Steve insisted on giving 90%. The trainer was furious as it messed up his figures. "You can't possibly mean that?" he fumed.

"I do! Mandy is my best friend too!"

Some might call it unhealthy that we spent so much time together, but for us it was perfect. All the while Steve was in hospital enduring his chemo sessions, I felt uneasy, edgy and, at times, fearful that *She* was 'preparing me for being alone' with these regular physical separations.

The three-day stretch in the Crypt was over again. I arrived early at 6.30 a.m. as Steve wanted to escape as soon as possible. The Royal Hospital building was foreboding with its gloomy grey walls and ghostly windows. I was sure that it was permanently overshadowed by black clouds, shedding tears of rain over all those who came and went through its doors. I arrived at the locked doors of Deansley ward, wet and bedraggled. I waited – my breathing rapid and shallow.

I discovered later that Deanesly Ward was built as a fever ward in January 1873. It was originally a separate building with no access from the main hospital. The Town Council, in 1882, fitted out the basement on condition they could send non-pauper small pox cases. To prevent the spread of infection, the doors of the fever ward were kept locked or secured by chains. Strange what you pick up!

You might think I'd be looking forward to the end of another chemotherapy session, and in some ways I did, but each time he seemed to get weaker, more desperate and quieter. I hated it and tried to do everything I could to cheer him up. But, when you think about it, his poor body had just been infused with deadly poisons whose role it was to attack the cells of the body, both cancerous and healthy ones! The onslaught is lethal. How does any cancer patient survive?

We settled, nevertheless, into our 'post-chemo' routine. I would collect Steve from the hospital and drive straight to Himley Hall fishing pool. In silence, I would bundle him up in layers and layers of coats, hats and scarves (even though it was now early summer Steve was always chilled to the bone). Some people, I am sure, would not understand why anyone could take such a poorly man to a fishing pond, instead of back home to a warm bed. But, it was Steve's life and Steve's choice.

"Come on, let's get you to the water's edge. Hope the fish bite today." I chirped. No answer. Steve just shuffled along and collapsed himself into the deck chair. I passed him the bag full of sandwiches (which he would just throw up later) and a flask of coffee (to make that task easier). I arranged his fishing tackle around him to be in easy reach for when he felt ready or able to start fishing, gave him a goodbye kiss and left him with his thoughts, just as he wished. I was to collect him in four, long hours.

I was always so downhearted at those moments. If Alex was with me, he too would wave at his daddy, a serious expression on his face, as if he also knew instinctively that daddy was not well and needed time alone. Trees surrounded the fishing pool, and often a mist would creep around the solitary shapes of those who sat beside it, waiting for the ripples to break its calm. When I looked back and saw Steve's hunched figure melting into the mist I shivered, fearing it would steal him away forever.

Steve was more forthright and down to earth about it. "I need to get the smell of the Crypt out of me – out of my body, my skin, my nose. Sitting by the fishing pool helps to blow it away. I don't want to come home straight away and bring that stench with me. I need to be alone. This is heaven compared to the Crypt."

I would sigh quietly and worry about leaving such a sick man outdoors at the mercy of the harsh elements. As I lingered by the car, I felt the chill wind biting my face. I needed to make one last check, so I tiptoed back to see if he was calling me to return. He wasn't.

Noticeably, few others braved this early hour beside the pool. I watched Steve from afar. His chest heaved considerably. Was he sighing? He breathed in the chill morning air, letting it clear his lungs. The effort made him lunge forward and cough. The men glanced at him, then at each other. They seemed keen to avoid small talk, I assume as it broke the peacefulness of nature around them, but I knew Steve would not mind. He had plenty of time, well, today at least. Yes, he was normally extrovert, talkative, the life and soul of the party

– joking and chatting with everyone, but these days, if I am honest – most days now – he had become monosyllabic and brusque with me (a side of his nature that I was not familiar with). He kept whatever reserves of energy were still left to him for talking and laughing with visitors. I understood, but I still wanted 'my' Steve back.

One afternoon, when I came to collect him from the fishing pool, I looked at him and nearly cried at the pitiful picture he presented – he was hairless, yellow and so incredibly thin. I wanted to wrap him in my arms and love the pain away. He looked so fragile and on the edge of life. There was so little to connect him physically with the man I had married.

I remembered the first time Steve took me fishing. He didn't catch anything at all, but my catch was worthy of a photograph. I needed two hands to hold the slippery carp. Steve had been so proud of me. I felt that ache of regret in my chest again. Would life ever be as it was before?

I stood beside him, looking into the black pool.
"I've had a funny day," Steve said with a big smile on his face. I was pleased that his mood seemed better suddenly.
"Go on…?"
"At half eight the warden made his rounds to collect the money for the day pass. I could hardly talk so I just nodded. He then asks me, 'Bacon butty order?' Now you know how I used to love bacon? Well, at this point I

felt that rush of sickness coming over me – my lips actually shuddered. I managed to swallow it down to reply, 'no thanks.'"

Steve held up his finger to signal 'give me a moment', and as if on cue, leaned over and threw up on the bank. I offered him a drink from the flask.

"Ta. Mandy, you'll never guess what happened next."

"No… carry on…" I urged him for the story, which I instinctively knew would become one he would enjoy repeating to friends.

"I was sitting here hardly able to move. I felt so shit. The pool was fairly busy today with some regulars and newcomers too. I don't really talk to them or engage 'cause whenever I go to speak I feel the urge to throw up again and I can't be bothered to be honest. I need all my energy just to sit here."

I was fascinated to have this insight of what he got up to when I was banished from the poolside.

"Anyway, I kept sniffing my hand to see if the hospital smell was starting to go, and this was interspersed, of course, with the compulsory throwing up into my sick bag. Well, it was bad timing on behalf of these two guys, who I think were looking for the best fishing pitch. I always choose this spot here as it's the quietest and no one ever sets up next to me. Well, these two guys were staring at me for ages and they finally waltzed over, with all their gear, to take up the spot just past me to my right. As they passed behind me, giving me a wide berth, I started to retch. The one guy scoffed and I heard him say,

'Bloody skinheads shouldn't be allowed to fish here. Disgusting behaviour!' And his mate whispered back,

'Yeah, I think we should report him. Bet he's taking drugs!'"

"If only they knew," laughed Steve, "Bloody ignoramuses, but it did make me chortle… and then, and then," Steve could hardly contain himself, "The first guy said, 'He looks dangerous to me. Maybe we should move further away.' And, they did." Steve was shaking his head, "Me dangerous… in this state. I couldn't stand up to swing an arm to swat a fly, let alone a person. Daft buggers!"

What had those guys seen to make them think those awful things about Steve? I took a step back and tried to look through their eyes. I started to smile.

"What? Why are you smiling?" Steve asked

"I get it. I get why they might have said those things. Think about it – you are bald – shaven headed in their view – wearing dad's donkey jacket and you've got your Doc Martens on – you do look like a stereotypical skinhead, who's drunk too much!"

Steve just huffed.

The pile of vomit was still on the bank beside him. Steve scuffed some soil over it as best he could. He grinned up at me, his eyes twinkling. Yes, he still had those mesmerising eyes.

"Well there's some more of the cancer out of me!" he said. His voice determined and sure.

"Ready to go home now?"

"Yeah, I'll live to fish another day!" he replied.

127

It was only a few weeks later that a similar case of 'mistaken identity' or stereotyping happened again. An elderly lady stumbled on the street in front of Steve. He had stepped forward to help, his protective nature coming to the fore as he tried to stop her falling over. Once he'd stabilised her, he bent down to pick up her shopping and apples that were rolling away down the pavement. The startled lady, who was obviously confused, just looked down at Steve's bald head, registered the rough-looking donkey jacket and 'bovver boots', then exclaimed in alarm,

"Oh, no! Leave me alone! Get away!"

It was so uncommon to see cancer patients in the street those days, so I guess it was an easy mistake to make.

Chapter 23: Me and Mrs Melly

Ever since banishing his morphine, Steve forced himself, every morning, to get out of bed and get dressed. Now he had gone one step further. He'd potter in the garden, record a mix tape of his music, wash up or insist on accompanying me to the park with Alex. It was certainly a slow shuffle, not unlike an elderly, worn-out man, but I never stopped smiling. It gave me such hope that he never stopped trying. We sat on the park bench, held hands and exchanged glances as Alex charged around like a box of fireworks. Sometimes, Alex would wave a stick in the air as if he was a knight attacking a huge fire dragon or other such creatures, in his quest to save the world.

"Life is for living, and *we* are going to live every moment," Steve said.

So we just kept walking the tightrope of our new life, knowing that the fathomless abyss was beneath us. 'Don't look down – place one foot in front of the other and keep your eyes on where you're going – straight ahead!'

When people in the street asked, "How are you?" Steve would always reply, "I'm okay. I just get on with it."

So determined was he to live his life (and get on with it) while he could, it often surprised me where he and his trusty friend – the sick bowl – ended up. Apparently, 'the sick bowl' was eager to help him rebuild a bright orange 1972 VW Beetle on our driveway. It also fancied taking a crack at a Sherpa Luton Campervan! It was clearly a sick bowl with a yearning for travel and adventure.

***

One morning, Steve staggered into the house, black grease smeared across his cheek and forehead, wiping his hands on a rag, "I give up. I just can't work out where the oil is coming from."

"I thought you were relaxing in the garden."

"Nah. Wanted to find that leak."

He sank down into the chair. I tried not to wince at the marks his oily overall was leaving on our settee.

He looked so dejected. He had spent hours out there yesterday, pouring over the Haynes manual and scrambling under the engine. Not, I suspect, what other cancer patients were doing, nor what Dr K expected him to be doing; his last words of advice to Steve had been, "Just take it easy. Your body needs to recover from each bout of chemo – get plenty of rest."

But not our Steve – that's wasn't his way! He was outside in the cold, lying on the floor, wrestling with the engine of the Campervan and its gear housing. Man versus machine. I looked at him and had to smile. Yes, he looked like a stick insect in a boiler suit, but his eyes shone with a passion for life.

"What?" he asked, catching my look of admiration.

"Just love you."

He rolled his eyes, "In that case ask Mrs Melly to help me find the oil leak."

Mrs Melly had been the previous owner of our home.
She was a grand old lady, who had herself worked as a
mechanic during the war. A 'first-rate' one, so the story
went. She had continued to service her own cars and repair them into her old age. A lady like that could definitely help Steve with his mechanical problem. Only
one small, 'incy, wincy' problem. She was dead.
"Go on Mandy. Please, for me," he pleaded.

What could I do? Refuse? Steve had been trying to
solve the problem for days. He always had such faith in
me, much more than I did myself, and he knew about
my 'ability' although it was not something I liked to
talk about very much. "Okay, but I can't promise anything."
Steve left me in the quiet as I settled down to meditate
and 'tune in'. I never really knew what I was doing. I
blundered on with only my instinct as my guide. 'Expect nothing and just see what happens' I told myself.

Blackness, nothing coming, then thoughts about the day
ahead… 'Okay, get a hold on this!' I chastised my wandering attention. I sent out a thought to Mrs Melly asking for her help. I waited, trying to relax, to find that
peaceful state which always precedes any 'image' or
'contact'.

Before long I was rewarded with a picture. It made me
jump though. I am always so shocked when my call is
answered. I never believe, right up until I get a response, that anyone is listening. But this time, something came though bright and clear, though I could not

recognise the image that I was 'seeing'. I began to re-produce it onto a notepad that lay nearby. I kept my eyes closed, the better to retain the image, and drew 'blindly' onto the paper.

"Steve," I called, still puzzling over the meaning of the picture I had just drawn.

Smiling, Steve's head appeared around the doorway, "Yeeess," he answered in a comedy high-pitched voice. I waved the drawing at him, "Makes no sense to me, but this – I am told – is what the underneath of the van looks like. And, Mrs Melly says you have been looking for one leak – you are wrong! There are two leaks. One is oil, but the other is brake fluid. The two leaks are converging so it looks like one – hence your confusion! Does this picture look familiar?" I passed my drawing into his eager hands. He stared at it with fascination, obviously making sense of my scribble.

"Ah, I see and yes, it makes perfect sense. I'm gonna go and have a look. Thanks, Mrs Melly." He called out to the air and raced off again.

I offered up my own thanks to her for making Steve's day, then sat and wondered about the nature of what had just happened. It wasn't the first time that I'd had this type of experience, but I could never totally believe it myself; I was never sure that it wasn't just the prod-uct of an overactive imagination. I wanted to under-stand what was happening. I wanted proof to go with Steve's faith in me.

A few minutes later I heard Steve cheering and hollering, "Yes! That's it. Mandy, I found the two leaks. Bugger me, I can't believe there was a brake fluid leak, but she was right. Thanks again!"

This uncanny ability to tune in to what you might call 'spirit', became part of our lives. I continually played it down, made excuses for its accuracy. After finding the needle in a haystack on more than one occasion I still trotted out the same excuses "It's just coincidence" "Another lucky guess" or "Must be intuition". But, as life went on, these 'psychic' moments became more prevalent and would sometimes have a direct impact on the people around me with whom I shared my insights. It felt like a double-edged sword – a burden and a blessing – to carry around with me. Steve had an unfaltering faith in me. He knew I would always do my best for others; that I would try to use my 'gift' wisely. I would not let him down.

Chapter 24: Special Bond

Twenty years later, we heard that a photograph of Steve was still hanging in the entrance hall of Wolverhampton Spiritualist Church, along with that of a small child. These two photos, displayed together, were kept as a reminder and as an inspiration to others of what is possible even when things look especially dark. I'd like to think that Steve's story has been told to others who were labelled 'terminally ill'. Many of them may still have died, but perhaps a few found Steve's story a source of strength that helped them fight on and overcome the disease that was once killing them.

Gary's parents carried him into the church. So frail and near death, yet everyone put on a brave face and discussed his forthcoming trip to Disneyland. Gary looked about eight years old. Steve sat and watched the scene, taking in the details before slowly moving towards the family group. Gary sat on a chair staring ahead, blank to all the commotion and concern around him. Steve approached him with a silly wave. Gary let out a tired sigh.
Sitting down next to him Steve leant forward and whispered something in his ear.
The little boy let out a laugh, causing his family to turn around, curious to see the cause of his laughter. Steve waved meekly to them. For the next ten minutes Gary and Steve giggled and whispered like two kids sharing a secret.

"It's so lovely to see him smile again," his mum confided to me, tearfully. "This is our last hope," her voice cracked as she choked back her sobs.

The doctors had diagnosed Gary with cancer of the spine and it had now spread to his brain. The family was counting the days he had left, which were 'not long now' according to his doctors. I placed my hand gently on her arm. Such a strong wave of feelings flooded over me that, for a moment, it felt like I was drowning. I had no words to offer her.

I could see that Steve was developing a special bond with this dying child. He always knew instinctively how to connect to children. It was one of the things I loved about him.

I sidled over to listen to their conversation. They were chatting about toy soldiers: how to paint them and make them look as good as new. They were so absorbed in this that they clearly lost interest in what was going on around them. Steve had found the hook, that got Gary chatting, that could lift him out of his darkness and discomfort. I watched as Doreen came over and lifted Gary onto her lap. She needed to make a physical connection with the child in order to start the healing. Steve stayed with them both, no doubt making Gary feel at ease until, as inevitably happened during a healing session, Gary fell into a peaceful sleep.

Once the healing session was over, Gary's dad picked him up to carry him back to the car. The boy stirred and looked around for Steve. They waved at each other,

"See you next week Gary, and don't forget the soldiers!"

So began a new friendship. Steve and Gary would meet up each week at the healing session. They were co-conspirators in the battle against the 'cancer army' invading their bodies. Those toy soldiers were such a good symbol for Gary to think about when he imagined fighting his own cancer.

As each week progressed, Gary got promoted up the ranks: starting at foot soldier, then progressing to sergeant, and onwards eventually to general leading his own army in the war against the evil cancer invasion. Together, and apart, Steve and Gary fought their battles hoping to be the victors in the war. There were setbacks: low blood count, another suspected tumour found lurking in ambush, blackout due to sheer exhaustion. All such setbacks trembled as they came under fire from their 'super anti-cancer armies!' Steve and Gary would avidly discuss tactics, new skirmishes to launch surprise attacks, and laugh at the pathetic attempts of the enemy to escape defeat.

Over the weeks we, the families and the healers, saw both our patients improve in demeanour and strength. But, always the question remained and hung in the air – would the doctors agree and give us the news – the confirmation of what we so hoped for?

Gary's mum could not contain herself, "It's a miracle! Gary's cancer is in remission".

"Brilliant news. Well done Gary!" beamed Steve.
The whole church was uplifted that day and we all left feeling so hopeful.
I so wanted Steve to have that same news – 'patience, have patience' I thought. 'Just keep doing what we are doing.' However, what happened next threatened to turn my resolve and positivity into dust.

Chapter 25: The Bell Tolls

"I don't know why I bother to make friends on Deansley ward," Steve complained. I did not want to be drawn into this difficult conversation. So I just nodded back sympathetically, not wishing to be swept into a spiral of pessimism and gloom. Inwardly I was praying that this time things would be different.

The smell hit us as we turned the corner. Steve visibly flinched these days and his face automatically turned a tint of green. I squeezed his hand as he shuddered. "Can't stand that stench," he mumbled, head down. "It's like dead people and smouldering dirty socks." That observation was not far from the truth. It triggered a grotesque image in my mind: of a monster – dark, slimy and grey with tentacle arms, long-fingered hands and twisted green nails reaching out to grasp and feed upon the life force of others. We walked, nevertheless, into its waiting embrace as if we had no choice.

"Morning Steve, Mandy. Are you ready for another bout?"
Steve grunted and shrugged in reply, but then found the good grace to smile brightly at the nurse… and pull her leg mercilessly. "Of course… I can't wait. I love it here being pumped full of radioactive chemicals and puking for England! I just keep coming back for more! Maybe after this bout I will glow in the dark and you can rent me out for Halloween!" He chortled at the nurse's expression and her uncomfortable body language.

I smiled to myself. Some of these nurses will never get Steve's dark humour, but humour was his defence, his lifebuoy in the fatal 'Jacuzzi of Despair'.

The nurse hesitated, but then smiled back. What else could she do? "Let's get you settled then."

Steve walked down the ward. I could see him ticking off in his head all the beds he has occupied over the months of coming here. I think he's been in every one! The nurse points towards the two-bedded side room. Steve stops abruptly and holds up his hand in protest. "This is your room," she beams.

I see her momentarily not as a nurse, but as the bed-and-breakfast landlady showing us our room for our weekend break away. I wish!

Steve peaks his head around the door. "Nope. I am not sleeping in that bed!" he declares emphatically.

Looking past his shoulder I totally understand. "Haven't you got another bed please?" I implore the nurse.

She looks confused, then frustrated, "No, this is the only one free."

My mind is sharply thrown back to the scene, only a few weeks ago, that played out in that exact same room when we were here last time.

Mike was so excited, "Steve I asked her to marry me and she said yes. I didn't want to wait any longer... because... you know why..."

"Congratulations, mate. That's fantastic news."

Steve had made several friends on the cancer ward over the months, and it was always good when their treatments coincided. It meant they could catch up on news and progress. Sadly a few had passed away, but those who survived became all the closer and seemed to give each other strength for the fight.

Mike was in seventh heaven.
"When is the happy occasion?" Steve asked.
"Sally is sorting out the date but we want to do the ceremony as soon as possible. Why wait?" he grins.

Things can change incredibly quickly on a cancer ward. Later that day there was a lot of flurry around Mike as he suddenly seemed to be experiencing breathing difficulties.
"Probably a reaction to the chemotherapy," Steve whispered to me. The curtains were still closed around him so we felt it more polite to keep our voices down.

Sally arrived with the vicar just as Steve was being taken off the ward for some tests. She waved and smiled as we shouted, "Mike told us he proposed. Congratulations!"

The following day when I visited I saw several 'Congratulations' cards alongside the 'Get Well' cards sitting on top of Mike's cupboard, but Mike wasn't there.
"You okay Steve?" I leaned over to kiss him.
He just looked at me blankly. Had I done something wrong?

"Oh bother! I forgot to get them a congratulations card."

Steve's voiced cracked as he said, "No, it doesn't matter now. He's gone."

"Gone home, you mean?" Something within me didn't want to comprehend the reality of the situation.

"He died last night." Steve turned his face away, as he swallowed and blinked back his tears.

It hit me hard. Odd, because I didn't know them well but something jarred. I started to ramble, "How can this happen? He was fine yesterday, so excited and happy. Oh my God, poor Sally, and his parents. Why? What happened? I don't understand… it can't be!"

Steve looked at me and took my hand. He understood my unspoken fears.

"I don't know really. They did manage to get married, though. An intense, quick ceremony at the side of his bed just a few hours before he went, died, you know."

'Is this how it might be for us? A sudden collapse and then it's all over'? My stomach churned and I felt sick.

"I thought Mike was winning. I thought he would beat this," was all I could say. In my mind I was comparing Steve to Mike.

He nodded, "Yeah, me too."

We sat there holding hands in silence for a while. Finally, my resolve kicked in and I landed a blow directly on the nose of that loathsome 'creature', self-doubt, just as he was beginning to wring his hands in glee, "Well you are NOT Mike!" I said firmly and confidently, "You are Steve and you will beat this, I am sure! Do

not let this affect you Steve, you will come through this
alive. No other outcome is possible!"
Steve weakly smiled. Momentarily I felt embarrassed.
This aspect of my character is scary – I take no prison-
ers when the going gets really tough, but I too was leading an army of a kind, and I had to be just as single-
minded in my own campaign as any other general on
the battlefield.
I rattled on for a while searching for something to talk
about that did not have the ring of death about it; that
felt more 'normal'. I wanted him to re-engage with his
future life, here with me. As usual, talking about our
son, Alex, seemed to do the trick. He smiled as I spun a
story for him, of all the antics Alex had been up to.

***

"No, I bloody refuse!" Steve's voice barked across the
ward. "My best mate died in that bed the last time I was
here! I *cannot*, will not, sleep in it."
I did not blame him as it was giving me the creeps too.
Logically I knew many others had probably been in that
bed since Mike died in it, but I knew it would not help
Steve's morale to sleep in the bed of his dead friend.
"Okay, okay," said the nurse. "Leave it with me and I
will see what I can do, but no promises as we are really
full."
"We will go for a drink," I suggested, "and come back
in about half an hour, an hour?"
"Alright. See you in an hour."

When we returned, bless them, they'd found a way around the problem. Steve was given another bed later that day.

Chapter 26: Foiled Again

I sighed. "Steve you can hardly stand. What makes you think you can start fencing yet?"

"Well, we can at least go and suss out the club."

I felt this was a bad idea. What would I do if Steve collapsed? He was so weak, especially after that last bout of chemotherapy.

Nevertheless, we arrived at Wolverhampton Fencing Club at 7 p.m. I had secretly telephoned the chairman earlier to 'put him in the picture' about Steve. The club members greeted us with smiles and Steve with encouragement.

"Would you like to do some fencing this evening, Stephen?" Lord David Falcon Stewart, the fencing coach, asked in his polished, proper English accent. I knew Steve wouldn't be able to resist as he glanced at me waiting for my agreement.

"If you feel up to it?" I held my hands open and shrugged indicating 'it's up to you'.

"Yeah, why not – no point waiting around. You never know if I will ever get this opportunity again."

I winced inside, "Of course you will. If you enjoy it, we can come every week."

David helped Steve into a fencing jacket. It hung off his bony shoulders and swung like a loose sack around his puny chest. The fencing mask proved another problem as it wobbled on his thin, bald head, but Steve was prepared,

"Hold on… I have a woolly hat in my coat pocket. I can use that underneath the mask."
Perfect snug fit – he'd been thinking ahead of course!

David began taking him through the basic stance and moves. I looked on. Steve was glowing with the pleasure of just being here – after all it was the first step to achieving one of his biggest dreams. But I became increasingly anxious, watching his legs wobble and his knees sinking under the stress of that additional weight and the effort of the basic moves. After only a few minutes he had to sit down for a rest, but he was not daunted.
David turned his attention to the other students, coming back regularly to check if Steve was ready to continue. That evening, he was probably on his feet for no more than five minutes, but we were there right to the end. Steve was completely involved (in his mind) – absorbing all the tuition he witnessed.

I realised that it would be a long time until I could leave him alone at the club. He was just too ill and his body unpredictable. So realising the truth of the old adage that 'if you can't beat them, join them', I too decided to take up fencing. Every week (except chemo weeks) we went along to the club. Steve soon became well known. Not because he was the 'poor bloke with cancer', but because he was such a natural, a quick learner with a real aptitude for this sport, and soon all the rest were lining up to fence him!

David and Steve got on exceptionally well, despite Steve challenging him continually and 'interpreting' his formal instructions out loud. For example, David would explain, "On my absence of blade…" and Steve would retort, "'On your absence of blade'… what the hell does that mean? Oh, you mean when you move your sword… like this…"
David would sigh, a little exasperated at times, but I think he saw something special in Steve so never took offence. He just patiently continued the tuition.

Steve's fencing style was often unorthodox, but he was able to spot gaps in other people's defence, and on those days when his strength increased, so did his scores and the tally of matches he won. No one could believe that such an ill man would attempt to fence; most of the time he could barely stand. He was driven by such a powerful determination though. I knew this and was thankful that he'd found a physical challenge that could both draw him on and in a strange way lift him up too, despite the extreme exertion it required. This was Steve's sport, his calling in some ways.

Each year the club had its own competition. Steve entered (wearing his woolly hat) and won every one of his matches – making him club epee champion. It was unbelievable. Step one on the road to him becoming a fencing champion.

Through my mind passed the consoling thought that even if he did not beat the cancer in the end, well at least he would have realised one of his life's ambitions. Fencing champion!

As if he read my mind, he turned to me and said, "Well that's club level. It's a start but I mean to go on and be British Champion." Of course, what did I really expect? Nothing less than the best. It struck me then that Steve was someone who needed goals that were really positive; things he could achieve; rather than things he must avoid – like dying. He wanted to be British Fencing Champion; he wanted to grow old with me; he wanted to see his son grow up. His willpower, these days, seemed to be forged of steel, like the epee he fought with. So, would it cut through everything that got in the way of those ambitions?

Steve was still three-quarters of the way through his chemo treatment plan when David put Steve's name forward for selection to the following year's training course with the Centre of Excellence for Fencing. If he was accepted, he would be fencing with the best in the country. This was a boost for us both – that someone else believed Steve would not only beat the cancer, but be fit and good enough to fight at that level next year.

To enter competitions at County level, however, Steve needed new equipment.

David explained why, "During the 1982 World Championships in Rome, Smirnov was fencing Matthias Behr of West Germany. Behr's blade broke during the action, and the broken blade went through the mesh of

Smirnov's mask, through his eye orbit, and into his brain. Smirnov died nine days later."

Smirnov's accident was the driving force behind the significant improvement of safety gear in fencing. Maraging steel blades (instead of the carbon steel ones of the day), Kevlar in the jackets, and masks two to three times stronger than the one he wore, all came about because of his death. I did not hesitate; I called Leon Pauls in London and ordered the new gear straight away – I had to keep 'my Steve' safe!

I remember one evening we had a visiting club come to ours in Wolverhampton. Some friendly matches were scheduled. Steve entered his first sabre competition. Sabre is not like the gentleman's sport of fencing (where only certain target areas are allowed and rules of etiquette apply); sabre fencing is more like 'no holds barred'; imagine Burt Lancaster in *The Crimson Pirate* meets Antonio Banderas in *The Mask of Zorro*. Steve was in his element – leaping about, slashing and hacking his opponent who repeatedly cried out with the pain of being hit. Needless to say, Steve won. He smiled at me as his opponent staggered away clutching his arm, complaining loudly about the injuries he'd sustained. Poor man, I could even see blood seeping through his white jacket!

"Steve you really hurt that guy!" I whispered through gritted teeth.
"Yeah I know. I love this sabre – it's a real man's sport! Anyway, he deserved it."

148

Surprised at Steve's attitude I glared at him, "What?"
Steve pulled me to one side out of view of the others.
"Look." He rolled up his jacket.
"Oh, Steve!"
His side was crisscrossed by angry slash marks – welts
of throbbing pain. A surge of empathy ran through me.
"Yeah… he came in so hard. That's why he always
wins – brute force. The other fencers hold back as
there's no need to hit so hard; it doesn't win you the
points. I was warned he does this, though. He's a mean
bugger, even with the older members, and I thought it
was time that he had some of his own medicine. It was
bloody painful, but I wasn't going to let on that he had
hurt me. Look at him now – doesn't like it when it happens to him!"

I'm not one to gloat at the pain of others but on this occasion I really did applaud what Steve did to that guy.
He deserved what he got, and I hope that it taught him a
lesson. Perhaps someone also told him that he'd received his thrashing from a cancer sufferer.

Looking back, I think fencing was like a 'double-edged
sword' for Steve – it used up a lot of his energy, sapped
him of the physical strength that he needed so badly
but, at the same time, it infused him with a lust for life
and vision for the future.

Chapter 27: Following in His Footsteps?

I sat next to the bed where Steve slept, my hand on his sleeping form, and gazed around the Crypt – a familiar place now. It was clinical, uninviting, and functional. Was that intentional? Everything seemed white. I remember white: white walls, white uniforms, white bedclothes, but I wonder, with hindsight, whether my memory has played tricks on me. Surely it wasn't all white, but painted in hospital green or yellow? It was certainly full of tangible emotion; on bad days, I picked up the echoes of the ghosts of grief, sorrow and fear. Everything would merge into one complete white environment. It felt like I was partly in an alternative reality, surrounded by white astral beings all closing in on me. But, I wasn't afraid; it was comforting.

I looked down at Steve's taut face, the skin stretched across his cheeks, and his sunken eyes. The clashing of fencing foils seemed so far away now – how quickly things change. The smell of Deansley ward was distinctive, repulsive, but my mind has blocked out the detailed memory so that now I can't even describe what it smelt like. I just know that I hated it.

"If it's washable, wash it!" Steve pleaded. The slightest whiff of 'that smell' from the Deansley ward days, even weeks after he'd worn or used something there, would set Steve off retching and reaching for a sick bowl.

I sensed movement behind me and turned to watch as a family I'd not seen before slid quietly onto the ward and sat around another sleeping form. The young woman looked about my age and the older woman with her must have been the mother of the lad in the bed. They glanced over and we shared that knowing, supportive nod.

"Hello," the older woman offered.

"Hi. First time?" I asked.

She looked towards her son, smiled weakly then walked over to me. Standing at the end of Steve's bed she lowered her voice, "No, second time."

"This is Steve's 10th treatment. He's doing great."

She seemed so sad, as if her son had already died. "Yes, we thought that about our Rick. He was doing great, but we're back again."

She sat down beside me and stared straight at me as if searching for an answer. Her eyes looked red and swollen as if they had been drained of tears. "Won't be long now the doctors say. He seems peaceful enough."

It was too much to bear, "But you mustn't give up hope. Who is his doctor?"

"Dr Lewis. A lovely man. Rick likes him."

What should I do? Should I say anything? I looked over to Rick's bed.

The woman continues, "Sorry, my name is Lily and that's my daughter-in-law, Donna. I have a lovely grandson, Mark. Cheeky like his dad was when he was little."

"How old is he? The son?"

"Mark's seven."

My thoughts travelled to our little Alex. He wasn't allowed to visit his dad as no children were allowed on the ward. I had started to see a change in Steve's attitude towards Alex. For most of Alex's life his dad had been in the hospital or at home in bed unable to play with him or carry him. Alex spent hours with my parents and had bonded well with my dad. I had caught Steve looking at them several times recently; it was a wistful look that said so much about Steve's longing to be a father to his son. Even now, so many years later, the memory of it brings tears to my eyes. It should have been Steve, who tickled Alex making him giggle uncontrollably. It should have been Steve who held his hand for those first tentative steps. It should have been Steve to whom he ran for comfort when he trapped his finger in the kitchen door. My dad was acutely aware of all this and tried his best to make Steve the centre of Alex's attention when he was home from hospital. But the memory of those first words still hung in the air when Alex had turned to my father and said, 'Dad'.

I looked over towards Rick. I wondered how many people had sat on this seat worrying if the person they loved would recover. Gradually losing belief in a shared future? I wanted, I needed Rick's mum to be more positive, to not abandon hope.

"Don't give up. He's young and strong."

"Well," she paused, "We've been where you are, believing he was getting better. He made a full recovery, so they said. Then it came back, fiercer, quicker and more vigorous than before. I hope it doesn't happen to you. There's no hope this time for Rick."

Tears threatened to pool in my eyes. I swallowed deeply to stop the sudden surge of raw emotion as she continued,

"Rick's tired. It won't be long. I worry for Mark and Donna now. How do you explain it to a child?" Confronted with the fragility of life and the nightmare of loss, I was conflicted. I was eager to offer comfort, yet afraid of stepping too close in case I invited similar devastation.

I couldn't answer her question. Selfishly my thoughts were back with my own son. At least Mark had known his dad for seven years. What if the same happened to Steve? Would I accept it? I shook my head. No, inside I knew this was different. It had to be different. I needed it to be different. Lily said nothing more. We sat in the silence.

Donna came over. I liked her immediately, even though we didn't talk much that day. A week later I was wandering around the newly built supermarket near Wolverhampton's Spiritualist Church, and there was Donna. We recognised each other and after a little hesitation we swapped phone numbers. I must admit that part of me resisted, irrationally fearing that sharing a friendship might mean that we would share the same fate: Steve would follow Rick's decline, or would 'give up' like Rick had. I cast those awful thoughts from my head and let my instinct guide me. There had to be something I could do. I needed them to be positive. He was too young to die – *they* were too young to die.

"Rick's out of hospital now," Donna said as she opened their flat door to me. "He is quite perky and seems a bit stronger."

Relief flooded through me. I was so thankful to hear that, for reasons I just couldn't explain to her.

"You okay with dogs?"

I nodded as I entered the dimly lit lounge. Six four-week-old Rottweiler puppies dominated their flat. Playful little creatures with a protective mother who surveyed me cautiously.

Rick was slumped in a chair, all his attention focused on the game he was playing with one of the little pups. It was jumping up excitedly to attack his hand, and with each failed attempt Rick tweaked its tail or patted its head to give it more encouragement. When he turned to me I saw a spark in his eyes, a shade better than the expression I'd seen him wear in hospital just a short while ago.

"Aren't they great?" his voice croaky and his breath shallow, "Bella's a good mum – a natural with them."

He began coughing and Donna quickly brought over the bowl. I looked away. Things were clearly not that great.

"Steve loves dogs too," I said. I felt awkward in their home.

What did I have in common with these two, apart from the cancer? Steve was the talker, the 'life and soul of the party', not me. I wished he was here with me. Most people, even those who know me well, would say I am a confident person, but I have always been nervous about meeting new people in new situations. I get tense, and sometimes I don't know what to say and, when I do speak, I struggle to form my words coherently. At moments like that I feel like I did as a small child watching the elegant, lithe-limbed girls do their ballet solos while I stomped behind them in the chorus, or when well-spoken, articulate people asked me a question clearly and confidently and all I could do was mumble back my reply becoming more acutely aware of my Wolverhampton accent with each word I uttered. Years later, when I was in secondary school, my father had the brilliant idea of paying for me to have private public speaking lessons. My tutor helped me to overcome my self-consciousness about my local accent and gave me the confidence to even volunteer to read out in school assemblies. However, occasionally the old Mandy – with her lack of self-confidence – returns for a visit.

My mother, I believe had the same struggles. I noticed, as I was growing up, that she would shy away from some people and then be a lively extrovert with others. Even now she still covers her mouth with her hand when speaking to strangers, as if she is afraid to be heard.

"Most people make me feel inferior," she told me once. It makes me sad as she has nothing to feel inferior about. She has overcome so many obstacles in her life, is so talented and admired by so many people for her friendly, helpful attitude. I am so grateful to both my parents.

As I grew up, I was keenly aware of my own shyness but I didn't want to miss the opportunity of meeting people or to allow my own feelings of inadequacy to limit me. So, I forced my timid voice to speak up; I smiled and trusted that people would find me as engaging as I found them. I picked up a valuable lesson from Steve and how he interacted with people, that everyone has something to say – some unique outlook on life, a cherished hope, a daring ambition – you've just got to look for it.

Donna disappeared into the kitchen. Rick and I filled the ensuing silence by focusing all our attention on the puppies, laughing at their antics as they tore around the lounge.

"So, Steve doing well?" Donna asked as she handed me a coffee.

"Yes," my enthusiasm overcame any inhibitions, "Everyone says he is looking better, stronger. I think he is beginning to beat it."

I felt a twinge of guilt. Rick was tired; he had overcome it once before. Would Steve be able to keep fighting if he was in the same situation? I was sure he would. Rick was as thin as Steve, but the air around him was thick with despair, helplessness.

Donna sat down next to Rick and squeezed his hand. She said, "We've been thinking about it."

Rick nodded to her in agreement.

"Steve really left an impression on Rick."

Rick joined in, "He is so damn positive. He makes me laugh how he curses at his cancer. He totally believes in this healing stuff."

I looked at Rick. I'd made the assumption that he was the sort who would ordinarily mock the idea of spiritual healing.

"We're not religious." I hesitated, "You don't have to be to... Doreen is lovely and everyone is so welcoming. We just thought it wouldn't do any harm, so why not try it?"

I'd never been asked to explain spiritual healing to anyone before. Steve had obviously told him something that had made him curious – or perhaps he was just desperate – so I took a deep breath and did my best to tell him our story so far. Rick never took his eyes off me. He listened intently without interruption.

Donna had settled herself onto the armrest beside him. She also payed close attention. I didn't want to give them false hope, but neither did I want to deny them the same opportunity that Steve had found. I was being my normal 'super-positive' self on the outside, but inwardly was thinking that even if it didn't cure Rick, it would help him feel calmer, more relaxed, so why not tell him about the healing? I couldn't guess whether Rick would ever accept healing himself, but I sensed he trusted Steve – who was just a 'normal' guy like him.

Rick winced and groaned as he was helped into the church and onto the cushioned seat waiting for him. His arms and hands were almost skeletonized. The texture and look of his skin reminded me of the photographs I'd seen of the Tollund Man, whose well-preserved body had been discovered buried in a peat bog. Rick's body was devastated by the disease, yet he persevered. He hardly spoke that day. Thinking back... all the courageous men and women I have had the privilege to sit with in the last few days of their life hardly spoke, but

157

there was always a moment when we made eye contact and I saw their eyes flicker with their suppressed emotions, desperation and fear. Those moments haunt me as I know I witnessed their raw helplessness as they faced, what they realised suddenly, was the inevitable outcome.

Doreen and Dot walked over to Rick, smiling, and began the process of healing, their gentle hands showing the way, their calm words offering encouragement. When it was over, Rick smiled at Donna, tears brimming in his eyes. He had felt something!

Rick visited the church many times before his death. I remember talking to Steve about it soon afterwards, "I think his body had deteriorated beyond the point of repair – past the point of reversal. Healers can only work within the natural law. In the end it was too late for Rick".

"He had the right 'positive' attitude in the end but it was already too late for him," he replied quietly.

I looked over at Steve and wondered if it would affect his resolve and spirit. He had convinced Rick to come for healing, yet... Rick had died.

Chapter 28: A Laugh a Minute

From the TV I heard the theme tune from that new soap 'Eastenders' ring out its first few notes,

"No, I don't want to watch that again – too depressing!" groaned Steve.

I sighed, as I fancied watching it. So many people were talking about it.

"I don't want to be another fly on the wall watching someone else's 'tragic life' unfold thank you very much," he grumbled. I suppose he had a point.

Soaps tend to focus on the negatives: domestic mishaps, arguments, betrayals, lies, crime... even murder. In fact all the things people come across from time to time in their lives, either close up or at a distance, but for the purposes of 'entertainment' these events are woven to-gether in one dense, sticky carpet of misfortune, which for some reason, we find compelling viewing. Holding that thought in my head, I argued:

"Well, that's partly what drama is for. People like to watch it and subconsciously feel better about their own lives. It's never half as bad as what's happening to the poor people in the programme."

"Huh, well it can't be healthy to take in all that negativity – don't you think?"

I looked at Steve knowing why he took that stance and that he wasn't going to budge. Well that was another one to cross off the list alongside the forbidden 'Hospital documentaries and dramas'.

"Okay, okay. So what shall we watch?"

Steve grins and waves a video case at me.

I saw the title. We'd watched it before – several times over I might add:

Here is a selection of just some of the 'comedy' programmes which we repeatedly watched:

- Blazing Saddles (the first film Steve took me to see – classic Mel Brooks stupidity)
- Fawlty Towers (a John Cleese classic)
- Black Adder (we loved the quick-fire wit and sarcasm)
- The Lenny Henry Show (great Midlands' characters)
- Porridge (Ronnie Barker at his best)
- Rising Damp (we all know someone like Rigsby)
- Spaghetti Westerns (even days after watching one, Steve would randomly chortle about some scene he'd just remembered)
- Airplane (puns and play-on words extraordinaire)
- Cheers (brilliant sarcasm and character interplay)
- Taxi (Danny DeVito – you've just got to love him… or not!).

They may look dated now, but this was still the 1980s and though there were fewer channels, the quality of comedy on TV was outstanding.

It became the norm in our house that if the TV was on, laughter filled the room. An atmosphere which I believe was a healing one. When we laugh I believe it releases certain chemicals (hormones and neuropeptides) into our blood stream, which relaxes our muscles and creates feelings of euphoria, love and happiness (like a joy

cocktail) which in turn aids the healing process of the body.
But on the other hand… there were times when it got too much:
"Oh no, turn off the TV. It's killing my stitches to laugh!"
"How do you kill stitches?"

I am sure we have all had those times when we laughed so much it hurts, but we can't stop. During those months following Steve's diagnosis, we actually had weekly occurrences of that! I am so thankful for all the comedians, comedy scriptwriters and producers out there for making Steve's sides ache, and giving me the pleasure of watching him smile and genuinely laugh while dying! Yes, I know I have a sick sense of humour sometimes.

We found our own source of amusement too: puns. We would land on a theme, then 'milk' it for hours.
"Morning sweetie," I pause briefly, as my brain latched on to the dizzying world of confectionery and all its possibilities, "I am wondering what sweeties would best describe you Steve: *smartie, werther's original, fisherman's friend?*"
"Not sour chew then?" replied Steve with no delay. Game on!
"Or *all sorts*, maybe *revels* or *ice breaker*, but definitely not *gobstopper* or *parma violet.*"
"*Cherry lips*?" he smirks and winks at me.
"Yes my little *bon bon.*"
"What about *love hearts*?"

"Or *malt... teaser*?"

"Oh… Will I get my *milky way* later on?"

"That was *boun... ty* get you thinking."

"Shall we get up today?" says Steve changing the subject.

"I suppose so, but when it comes to the *crunchie*… you are my *matchmaker* and *treats* are in order because you are just down my *quality street*."

"You *flake*!" he laughs, "Oh dear, no *roses*?"

"Yes please and some *black magic*."

"You're getting worse than me."

"Taught by a master, who has me wrapped around his *curly wurly*."

"Now, you are *butterkist*… ing me up."

"Groan, where's a *flying saucer* when I need one?"

"Did you remember to put the *milk bottles* out? Sorry, I am getting worse."

"Let's change the *topic*!"

"Yep worse. It's turning into a bit of a *marathon*."

At that time anything could set us off, and puns always make me smile in memory of those days. I know it's a cliché, but laughter is the best medicine and just because someone is seriously ill, even with a terminal diagnosis, it doesn't mean they can't still enjoy a laugh, a pun or a joke, even if it is that special black humour. Compassion and sensitivity are necessary, but laughing at life, to me, is essential.

Chapter 29: Dark Opening

As I write this today, I'm thinking back to when Steve's mum died. It's the anniversary of her funeral. She too died of cancer. It deeply saddens and confounds me that Steve's parents chose to keep their distance when Steve was so ill. Perhaps it was too painful to witness their son in such agony. I know I'm looking for excuses, as in truth I could never understand such a decision. But years later when Jean (his mum) was herself extremely ill, they chose to keep it quiet and retreated from contact with us. It was just their way I suppose. Everyone deals with illness in their own way. Jean was a pleasant woman; she had a jovial attitude towards life, but in the end – and who knows what the circumstances were that led to it – they stopped her treatment, withdrew fluids and increased the morphine. Sitting by her bedside, hours before she passed, she was unable to talk or move. I reached out to her with my mind, gazed into her eyes and I knew her spirit was at peace.
Had that happened to Rick too just before he died? I don't know.

***

Rick's was the first funeral I'd attended. It was traumatic.
Steve shook his head afterwards, "That's one funeral I'll never forget."
Rick had been buried in accordance with Jamaican traditions, as that was Donna's heritage.

"It was really hard on his son," I said. It was so harrowing to hear Rick's tormented son cry out at the grave-side, as he pulled towards the coffin that contained his father.

"I want my dad! I want my dad!"

His grandma, Lily, reached out to pull him back as the coffin was lowered. It was a futile bid to calm his sobs. Mark sought solace by burying his head in his mother's dress and flaying his fists against her. I held my breath, wishing to hold back the sobs, but the tears fell anyway. I didn't dare look at Steve. We held hands silently at the grave-side.

Four of the mourners took a shovel each, and reality hit home. In Jamaica the custom is that the men bury their own dead. 'Thud!' Thud! Thud!' echoed round the graveyard as the soil fell onto the oak casket. Each shovel full that dropped broke the silence with a doleful rhythm, until the task was done and the stillness returned. It seemed so final.

Rick's son looked at the pile of earth, his eyes red raw, straining to 'be a man' and not cry. Poor soul. 'Don't let that happen to my son' I prayed.

"You shouldn't have gone, Steve. Rick would have understood." I sat on Steve's bed, onto which he'd collapsed as soon as we got home. He looked tired and drawn. I couldn't ignore the pinched features and sunken dark-ringed eyes. How could I not see on Steve's face all the signs of the disease that had ravaged Rick before he died? Where was my handsome Steve, the one I was sure would return to me? "Try to get some sleep. Call me if you want me."

I know he didn't sleep but he needed time on his own. Rick had become a close friend; one more to disappear from the cancer ward. They were an endangered species. Steve was, now, the only patient still alive from the original ward intake of twenty patients onto Deansley.

I admit I was a little half-hearted in even trying to keep up contact with Donna afterwards and I believe she felt awkward around us, so inevitably the friendship dissipated. However, a few months later Donna and Rick were to become a talking point again.

"Steve, I had a dream about Rick. It was so real. He looked fantastic. Full of life, vibrant, healthy like we have never seen him." I faltered, "We were in a brightly lit hall and he called me over. He talked about Donna and asked me to give her a message."

"What was the message?"

"He said he wants me to tell Donna 'it's okay'. He wants her to be happy. Apparently she has a new boyfriend. This bloke was a friend of theirs, who really helped her after the funeral, and it's developed into a relationship. He is fine with it."

"Mmm, bizarre!"

It was bizarre because two days later I was going up an escalator in The Mander Shopping Centre in town and there was Donna passing me in the other direction. I jumped off at the top and hurriedly returned on the down escalator, wanting to catch her up. Instantly I knew the purpose of the 'dream'. Donna was embarrassed and tongue-tied at first. I felt as if Rick was there encouraging me to tell her. I had to pass on the message, didn't I?

I did.

I could see the shock on her face, but then the relief as she smiled and looked straight at me, "It's true, I am in a new relationship." She looked distant for a moment, "I hoped he wouldn't mind, but it's nice to hear it from someone else. Thanks for telling me. We will come round sometime and visit you and Steve."

I haven't seen or bumped into Donna since. I often wonder what she is doing now and what happened to their son, Mark.

Chapter 30: Notes and Crosses

I could feel the warm soothing heat through my blouse as I laboured over my art pieces, paintbrush in hand, in the pleasant sunshine of the back garden. I felt peaceful and content. I stood back to admire my handiwork. "Nearly finished!" I shouted to Steve whom I could hear moving around in the kitchen. We had less than four days until the fête and I had been amusing myself in a world of flowers. Getting inspiration from our garden, I had painted a whole array of different species, and at this moment was adding the final touches to the last piece.

The doorbell chimed. We weren't expecting anyone. "I'll get it!" Steve offered and shuffled to the front door, clutching his dressing gown over his bare chest. Through the glass porch he could see two young, clean-cut guys wearing business suits, white shirts and dark ties. They were smiling at him. Steve glanced at their telltale name badges.
In the past he may have turned them away, but today I heard him respond, "I think I know why you're here. We are in the garden. You are welcome to come in for a cuppa. But, just so you know: we don't believe in Jesus as our saviour." They weren't put off.

As they trailed after him from the hall into the kitchen, I heard one ask,
"Do you mind if we have a glass of water? We are not allowed caffeine or other stimulants."

I imagined Steve smirking to himself as he filled their glasses. Through the window I saw Steve pass them both a glass of water and put the kettle on for us. He led them to the backdoor. As they stepped into the garden all three held up their hands and squinted into the sunlight – momentarily blinded.

"Take a seat," Steve waved his hand to the other two deckchairs.

Steve sat down with a huge smile on his face.

The two guys stood motionless. They were staring past me. Their faces registering utter confusion.

I turned to look at what had them so spooked.

Ah, the crosses! That explained it. Behind me was my day's work. A sea of fifty-two white crosses all hanging by string fixed to the washing line with pegs, or hanging from tree branches. They swayed gently back and forth in the wind, impossible to ignore and confusing to behold no doubt. Steve had made each cross (7 inches long with a 3-inch crossbar) and painted them in gloss white for me. I simply decorated them with pretty flowers. I hoped to sell them at the church fete.

I surveyed the sea of crosses. To me, they looked amazing, almost alive, dancing in the breeze. But to unfamiliar eyes perhaps it had the look of a field of remembrance. Slowly, the two Mormon missionaries dragged their eyes away from the scene and conspired silently to say nothing about it.

"So where are you from?" Steve opened the conversation.

"I'm from America – Boston, and Philip is from the Netherlands."

"So what are you doing here?"

Bless them – on cue they went straight into their re-hearsed spiel, which was no doubt intended to lead us to 'redemption' but Steve was having none of that:

"No, tell me about you and how it works being a mis-sionary?"

"We're both serving two years on our mission to spread the word. I have nearly finished my service, and when I return I will go back to university and get married. We work in pairs all the time, rarely leave each other's side, but when I am reposted Philip will have another com-panion. We change mission companions around every four months. It's been an amazing experience, one I will never forget."

"Who funds you?"

"My community, the church and family back home."

"If you are moving around every few months, what happens to your living accommodation?"

"When I leave our accommodation another missionary will take it over, so the rent continues to be paid. Same with sharing our bikes."

"Do you get to see or do much in the countries you're in?"

"We have a disciplined daily schedule. We get up at 6:30 and go to bed at 10:30 every night. We agree not to date, flirt or even be alone with a member of the op-posite sex while we're on the mission. No TV either, just reading the scriptures and other religious books. Sometimes we listen to inspirational music. I know it sounds hard but it's been the best two years of my life."

I admired their dedication. No doubt they wanted to show us the 'true path' as they saw it, but they were respectful enough to not force their views. To be honest, we hardly spoke about religion with them; we just simply enjoyed each other's company. I believe, however, that we all have an eternal spirit (some call it a soul) which is our true selves and essence; and that the 'spirit of a person' can connect with the universal energy, the life force, God, One power or whatever you want to call it; and that we are all connected somehow spiritually, energetically and physically – hence more and more, I was trying to reach out and 'touch the souls of others' because when we really 'see' each other, there is no 'us and them', no separation or discrimination – we just 'are'. So many people hide their true, wonderful selves behind the masks they create and the roles they take on. I like to try to feel and see the real person.

We never saw the two missionaries again, but it was a pleasant afternoon and I enjoyed the insight into their life.

The following day, it was back to the Crypt.

When I arrived at visiting time, Steve was retching from the pit of his stomach, yet producing nothing. The stench of the place immediately hit my nostrils like smelling salts, and clung on like vine tendrils to a rendered wall. Was the smell from the ward or rising from Steve's body? I looked at the drip once more in his vein, pumping in the poison, and I felt helpless as I watched Steve visibly turning corpse white by the minute. We sat in silence trying to hold the moment at a safe distance. Yes, this is what we did, what we had to do, but it wasn't who we were.

The doctors came round to prod and poke. We listened without really paying much attention; on another level we knew they had nothing positive to report. Meanwhile my mind fell into its old tricks of conjuring up scenes of death and grief, rehearsing for a future that I was determined not to have. Tomorrow would I see a white sheet over Steve's head?

"They're gone," Steve's voice reached into my thoughts.

"Oh, good." I stammered and looked at my watch.

"You get back to Alex." Steve took my hand and repeated his ritual bedtime mantra to me, "I will feel better tomorrow!"

"I know!" I smiled, "Love you too."

As I walked away I had a nagging feeling something significant was about to happen.

***

When I returned the next day, Steve sprang up into a seated position in his bed – his drip down to its last few drops.

"You know when you disappeared yesterday?" he asked.

I nodded.

Steve seemed agitated. "I was thinking, we're a young married couple with a baby. We should be out on a beach with our son, flying kites, playing tag, that sort of thing. But here I am in this bloody prison, retching and puking my guts up, just hoping to survive another night."

"Okay," I was not sure where this was going.

"Remember the doctors had just gone?"

"Yes."

"They left my medical notes on my bed!" he declared triumphantly, "I read them from cover to cover, including all their side notes!"

Oh God, what had he read? What had they written? Had they told us everything? Had he seen the prognosis of just three months? I'd never told him about the three-months – if he found that and realised I knew but had not told him, would he ever trust me again? If he saw the prognosis would he believe it and give up now? In panic, I couldn't speak.

"Appears my cancer was first diagnosed as a 'nervous stomach'. Nervous stomach, my arse! Another doctor wrote suspected 'kidney stones' – okay, I'll give them that. Then surprise, surprise, tumours here there and everywhere."

Was Steve angry, pleased? I couldn't tell.

"But you were right, Mandy. Everything you said was in there." That was a relief, I suppose.

"Anything we didn't know?" I ventured (praying desperately that he did not say 'yes, I had three months to live!')

"Nah, don't think so. Just 'not responding to treatment', which we knew."

I squeezed his hand, "Well you are still here to prove them wrong."

"Yes…" he retched again, and threw up into the sick bowl, which I offered reflexively whenever I saw his stomach heave.

We locked eyes as he wiped his mouth and, in unison, we proclaimed, "There goes some more of the cancer!"

Chapter 31: The Walking Dead

Eve's nightclub in Wolverhampton 1982 – a young black man strutted his stuff around the dance floor, executing all the moves to Michael Jackson's 'Thriller', with complete precision and perfect timing. He reeled in my gaze like I was a sleeping fish; I was transfixed! He danced in front of one of the huge speakers. I wondered how it didn't deafen him to be so close to the source of the booming music. Occasionally he reached back and touched the speaker itself. Confused and strangely entranced, my eyes were locked on him. It was like I recognised something. A young Asian lad tapped him on the shoulder and signed to him. Of course, they were both deaf! They both looked in my direction so I signed,
'Hello, I like your dancing'. And thus started our wonderful friendship with 'Thriller Pete'.

In my first year of teaching deaf children, Steve and I had decided to start running the Wolverhampton Deaf Youth Club. We both had basic signing skills and felt it was something we could do together, hopefully making a difference to some of these children's lives.

'Thriller Pete' was the DJ for our first disco at the Deaf Youth Club. Everyone turned out, dressed up to the nines. Short skirts, makeup, slick jackets and ties. It was a fantastic night and the first of many. We would organise something different each week for the youngsters to experience. I remember another evening when our martial arts Aikido Club put on some self-defence training. The local press attended and caught Steve in action! We tried to run the youth club by involving the youngsters as much as possible in deciding the events and activities.

Pete helped out, often communicating for us when we got stuck. He became a great friend and I never thought that just a year later I would be giving an emotional, signed speech at Pete and Marie's wedding. It's hard to sign and brush away the tears. I am so sentimental!

We also attended many social events at the Deaf Social Club (for adults) and so many people in the deaf community came to know and recognise us. When I was pregnant with Alex we decided to hand over the running of the youth club to someone else, ideally someone deaf. Although it took a while to persuade him, Pete eventually became the Youth Leader.

Due to my pregnancy and Steve's subsequent illness, we had not been able or well enough to visit the youth club, the deaf social club, or see any of their members. We assumed that the word had got out and they would be sending Steve their best wishes.

One day on the way to hospital, we bumped into a deaf couple that we knew. They both stared open mouthed and didn't sign back in greeting. It was embarrassing as they just kept looking at each other. Was this a deaf culture thing? Were they under some misconception that it might be catching or something? What was it?

I asked if they were okay and Sylvia slowly signed,
"We thought Steve had died… or was dying!"
Ah, that explained it.
Her eyes were pleading with me to tell her otherwise
but she kept glancing at Steve and shaking her head.
Steve was obviously 'the dead man walking'!
I looked at him through their eyes and took in his ema-
ciated figure, his gaunt face and sallow skin. Poor
woman. I could see her shock. I suppose Steve did look
close to his own demise, but I was just so used to seeing
him that way now.
Steve laughed as usual and signed, "Nah, I'm still here.
I'm fine!"
From their faint smiles it seems they did not believe
him.

Steve and I enjoyed imagining the scene back at the
deaf social club: the grim fascination as they all discussed how Steve was holding on to life by his fingernails, while slowly turning into a zombie.
Needless to say it was the time before computers,
emails, and mobile phones so unless someone from the
deaf community actually found out where we had
moved, and came to visit us in person, the likelihood of
any further contact was small.
Seeing the extreme reaction of Sylvia and her partner
just reminded us of how awkward people could be
when confronted with serious illness and the spectre of
death. They were so uneasy.
This chance meeting, however, got us talking about the
future. Would I go back to teaching deaf kids? When

should we visit the deaf club? We knew that we both loved sign language and often signed to each other.

"I have that 'old irresistible pull' to be more involved in the deaf world – as if there is more for us to do there," I said

"What's stopping us?" Steve replied with a grin.

Chapter 32: Final Countdown

Steve had lived *well beyond* the three-month deadline that Mr Rogers had given me on diagnosis. Did I dare drop my guard? He seemed stronger, more positive, yet we had been here before and had reeled under the blow of the assertion that 'the treatment is not working'.

"Let's check your stomach today Steve."
Dr K silently prodded and rolled his hands around Steve's lower torso. He did not smile, but nodded. The examination seemed longer, more exhaustive than usual. I wondered what was going on. I held my breath. Dr K said, "The tumours *are* shrinking." He turned to look at me. "I am shocked. I don't know how. I've been an oncologist for many years. During that time, I have seen only a handful of what I would call 'miracles' and this is one of them. I'm very doubtful that the chemo-therapy *alone* has done this. Whatever else you are do-ing, Steve, keep on doing it because it is working!"
What can you say in response to a 'miracle'?
"You are winning Steve! It's official." I began to cry with tears of gratitude and sheer relief. It was like Dr K had lifted a great weight from my shoulders.
I was surprised that Dr K admitted that he believed that Steve's recovery was a miracle and that other factors were certainly involved, but I wholeheartedly agreed with him.

In subsequent years every medical person we have spo-ken to has said that they too can't understand how Steve recovered. Thirty years later, I am elated that science

178

has now started to explain some of that early 'miracle', giving substance to our belief that his recovery had, indeed as Dr K said at the time, very little to do with the chemotherapy guesswork. We worked in blind faith and complete conviction all those years ago, to beat that cancer, just knowing that we were doing the right thing. I am certain that our super-positive attitude, all the laughter we enjoyed, and our belief in a healing power (both our own body's power to heal from within as well as the contribution of the universal healing power) were, and still are, vital to enable us each to live fully and to regain and maintain our health, even in the face of serious illness.

"So that's it? Steve is getting better, he is beating it?" asked my dad with tears choking his voice.
"Yes, Steve is beating it!"
"Amazing."
"Unbelievable… " We got used to hearing these words of response from everyone we told.

On 25th September 1986 Steve was officially in remission. It takes around nine months to grow a new baby in the womb, Steve took nine months to grow a 'new body', one free of cancer! All he had to do now was keep it that way, and not allow the cancer to return! Could he do it? How would we do it?

Chapter 33: One Last Secret

Keeping secrets – it's not something I like to do as a rule (especially from Steve), but this one was the cause of much excitement. I had to keep pushing away the thought that it could all backfire and end in disaster. We had tickets for a 60s evening taking place at The Maltings, a community centre in Wolverhampton. We were going with Paul and Angie, to celebrate Paul's birthday.

Steve had been out fishing with Paul all day – unsuccessfully I might add – and they both returned to our house smelly, cold and miserable.

Paul whispered to me, "God Mandy, Steve wanted to come home half way through the day. The fish just weren't biting at all. Bloody typical eh! I really had to work hard to keep him out in the freezing cold. He must have thought I was really mean insisting we stay, but I managed to persuade him."

"Thanks, Paul, you are a star!"

"See you later then. Make sure you're in your glad rags!" Paul called cheerfully as he left to get ready for 'his' party night, "Meet you in the car park at 7.30."

"I don't really feel like going out tonight," Steve said quietly.

How did I play this one? Keeping my fingers crossed I offered "Nor me… we could phone them and cancel I suppose?" This was a gamble and I knew it.

"Hmm… but… Paul's been so good to us, we can't let him down," he replied.

I sighed dramatically, "Oh I don't know what to wear though. I don't have anything 60s style. Shall I be different and wear my dirndle dress?" I knew Steve loved me in my German national costume.
"Yeah! Be different."
I can't believe it myself, but mischief got the better of me: right before leaving I questioned him again "Are you really sure? We can call them and cancel if you want – if you are too tired. I'm sure they would understand."
"No, no we are ready now and it might be fun."
Mmm, I thought 'Does he know? Is he just playing along?'

I had had an insanely busy day, getting everything organised. And I was just hoping that it would all go to plan.
The car park was full, but luckily Steve did not recognise any of our friends' and family's cars. We walked with linked arms, the four of us, up to the community centre front door. Angie was chattering away to distract Steve and also to deflect attention from my sudden nervousness. "Great hunter-gatherers you two are! No fish for our supper," she teased.

As we reached the door, my sense of drama returned, "Are you sure we have the right place? Or day?" I asked with an air of uncertainty. Inside, everything looked empty and dark. "Yeah," mused Paul fishing out his ticket to check.

Like some rehearsed choreographed dance Paul, Angie
and I moved in unison to let Steve take the lead. He
reached for the front door. It was unlocked.

We followed him inside.

"Strange," said Steve, "it's so quiet."

"Let's check inside there first… maybe there's another
room running off it?" I hesitantly suggested, sounding
unsure myself.

Steve reached forward and pushed open the door.

He stepped into the dark hall with us three close behind.
Too close as it turned out.

The lights suddenly blazed on, and a unanimous chorus
of cheers, and laughter broke out. Steve stepped back in
utter shock trampling on the three of us behind him. We
all nearly fell on top of each other. Staggering to keep
our balance and trying not to lose shoes in the melee,
we quickly adjusted to the light and took in the scene
before us.

"Sorry, sorry," I heard Steve say apologetically, turning
to leave. I realised in an instant what was happening.
Steve thought we had accidentally gate-crashed someone's surprise party.

Laughing, I turned him back round to face everyone.

Voices filtered through the cheering and clapping,

"Congratulations Steve!"

"Well done, mate."

"You did it. Fantastic!"

Everyone wanted to tell him what a marvellous thing
he'd done. It was overwhelming.

Steve shook his head, not knowing how to react. He
was so bowled over.

I gently pushed him through the crowd, tears beginning to threaten my makeup. I welled up and gave into the mascara smudges, as I heard Steve's awe-struck voice, putting names to the faces of those who had come from near and far to be with him this night.

Some he'd seen that week, some not for months, others not for years – but they all meant such a lot to him. Friends, family from the UK and abroad, neighbours, colleagues, nurses, doctors – over a hundred people, all of whom had been touched by Steve's story and contributed in some way to his success. Back patting, hugs, kisses, words of love cocooned him and I cried in joy and gratitude.

"You really didn't know or guess?"

"No, I honestly had no idea."

"I thought you may have come across one of the invitations in my handbag?"

"No. What invitations?"

I showed him a 'Steve's Surprise Party' invitation which was printed with the words '*An Inspiration To Us All*' underneath the date, place and time. It looked so much like the one in his hand printed '60s Evening'.

"Yes same printing, the same style, except there were only four copies of that bogus '60s Evening' one, and a hundred and fifty of the real ones!" I laughed, a profound relief flowing out of me.

The band began to play and the lady started to call everyone up for the first barn dance. Steve had always enjoyed barn dances and it had seemed the best way to get everyone of all ages meeting and laughing.

"Ah, now I know why you wore your dirndle dress – most appropriate!" smiled Steve.

The evening passed in a whirl. I felt as if we were both talking and smiling non-stop. Some say it's impossible to describe love; you can't see it, you can only feel it. Well, I had the privilege of seeing the effects of love that night. So many selfless and caring friends and family had helped to bring the surprise party idea into a reality. That group of people showed such unconditional love to me and Steve that night. It was deeply personal but also tapped into something much broader and higher – the love of human souls for each other, in times of joy and pain. It was wonderful and I wish I could just bottle it up and send it to people when they need it.

As the evening drew on, Steve and I stepped to one side for a while.
"Steve, is there anything you would change?"
"Well, I could have done without the pain, but I suppose, we achieved the impossible."
"So if you could go back in time and not have the cancer at all, do you think you would?"
Steve looked to the ground, weighing up his answer, "No, I wouldn't change it. The experience has given us so much, taught us so much… for the better. Life is great. I don't want to waste my life or get caught up in things that don't matter."
"Yep, life is for living. So what are we going to do next?" I asked.
"Fly?"

Chapter 34: Flying High

"Pearls symbolise tears and wisdom," Jean, my mother-in-law explained, as she placed the gift box in my hands at the party.

I always thought pearls were for old people, but this was a beautiful necklace which I would, of course, always treasure.

"This is too fiddly!" Steve complained as he finally fastened the delicate clip securing the pearls around my neck. "Hurry up. I have to be there in half an hour!"

It was another milestone for Steve. My gift to Steve at the surprise party was a voucher for his first ever flying lesson, so he could take to the skies and fulfil another of his boyhood wishes.

So, that chilly November morning we arrived at Halfpenny Green Airport for his Cessna flight training and first flight. Last time I was here was on 28th August 1972 watching the air show with my parents, when the aircraft piloted by Prince William of Gloucester, a cousin of the Queen, crashed into a hedge just beyond the airfield's boundary soon after take-off. He and the co-pilot died trapped in the flames. It was horrific. Flashes of the incident came back to me now – the plane plunging to the ground, the wide-eyed gasping of the crowd, shouts of panic and distress, the emergency vehicles scraping past the parked cars in the narrow country lanes. I recall, that for weeks later, one of the wings from the fallen aircraft lay in the garden not far from where we'd been viewing the display.

A smile stretched across Steve's face as soon as we glimpsed the waiting Cessna 182.

"Bi-yee," Steve shouted as he bounced off like an excited kid following his flight instructor. Richard, our video man, was at their heels recording the precious memories. He was a friend from our school days, and had filmed the surprise party for us. It was his idea to take footage of Steve up in the air as a coda to the film he'd made already… showing Steve's ascent into deep-blue sky of the future.

Alex peered at the posters on the wall. He liked exploring the waiting room, but he soon clambered on the chair to look out of the windows and point excitedly at the planes.

I joined in, "There's daddy. Look. He's climbing into the blue and white plane." My heart was thumping. After all we'd been through, what if his plane crashed? I know, stupid thoughts. "Daddy will be fine Alex. Look, look he's taking off. Wave to daddy."

I contemplated our family motto 'Believe in yourself, and everything is possible'. What had we learned this far? How had it affected Alex? What else might be out there waiting for us? What did we wish or want to achieve next? We had overcome impossible odds. Steve had survived his death sentence. So why not aim high?

Alex clung on to me, struggling to keep an eye on the plane as it flew out of sight into the clouds.

I felt a tug, then heard a snap. I looked down at Alex – he was held tightly in my right arm, his legs clasped around my hips as he struggled and pushed up on me to see more. He did not mean to do it. We were both stunned for a moment by the unexpected symphony of tap dancing pearls, cascading across the floor.

He grinned his daddy's grin, as we both realised what had happened.

I sprang into action. "Quick Alex, grab them!"

I put him down on the floor and frantically scrabbled around on my hands and knees. The pearls had scattered in all directions.

Alex slowly walked among them, carefully picking one up to scrutinise it then throwing it back down on the floor. He laughed as it bounced and rattled to its resting place. A new game?

I managed to find most of the individual pearls and put them in my pocket, but some of the escapees are probably still there hiding under the skirting boards.

"Oh, well mummy's pearl necklace has gone Alex. Huh, I suppose that means no more tears for us!"

Steve returned triumphant. "It was brilliant, Mandy. He let me take the controls. It was great to feel the plane respond to me." His voice quivered with excitement, "I loved it."

Alex handed his daddy our present.

"Shall I open it now?" Steve asked.

Alex nodded eagerly.

Steve ripped off the wrapping and held up the toy Cessna. With his strong arms he hugged us both.

"Daddy's plane. Daddy's home." Alex said simply, firmly and with absolute knowledge.

Tears rolled down my face. Yes, that was so true, Alex. Daddy was back for good.

Epilogue

Steve and I went on to both work as fully qualified sign language interpreters, disability awareness and mindset trainers, and to run several businesses together (including a dog grooming salon). We spend day and night, work and leisure times with each other. Some ask, 'How on earth can you manage to spend all that time together?' I, for one, would not change it. We still aim to continually support, trust and believe in each other.

Has life been all plain sailing since? Hell, no! We have had many challenges in the family, including accidents and ill health, e.g. MS, car accidents, a serious heart condition. And, each time, we dusted off our PLAN, discussed amendments and moved forward into a better future.

One challenge was being told that Steve was infertile. We found a way around that (where there's a will there's a way!) and now we have three grown-up children – Alexander, Dean and Renate.

Okay… so one of our children happens to be deaf-blind and autistic; another is partially deaf and the third is dyslexic. However, by seeing the great potential in each child first and foremost, before their so called 'disability', a world of fantastic opportunities for fun, love, growth and creativity opened up for us all! I am not saying it was easy, without incredible stress or sleepless nights. It did, for sure, have an effect on our health, but it also gave us the tools and experiences necessary to help others turn around their own challenges, stresses, fears and frustrations so that they too could live a life that is enriching beyond measure.

After Renate was born, we decided to buy and convert an old Victorian primary school in Shropshire into a home. In the beginning of this adventure we were all living and sleeping in one classroom surrounded by building materials, dust, dust, and more dust! The kids loved the fact they had their own playground complete with netball court markings on the tarmac.

Our love of the countryside led us next to buying a small holding on the Welsh border. The five of us spent 14 years here with our Soay sheep, chickens, our short-haired English collie Fritz, and tabby cats Acuba and Kitana. We home schooled Renate there until she went to college.

Steve and I now enjoy a sea view every morning (fulfilling yet another dream when we relocated to the Devon coast five years ago).

'Ooby-dooby' wise? Yes, those experiences still keep occurring! I realise looking back that I find myself, much more often than others do, in situations (too numerous to mention here) whereby someone is near death. I sense what is happening and seem able to communicate with their spirit. I am in the right place at the right time, perhaps? I feel honoured to do this – to help them in my role as 'spiritual nurse' or 'midwife' to the afterlife.

One such occasion was when a man was involved in a hit and run car accident. He'd been thrown into the air and landed on his front. Steve immediately pulled over and I ran over to the injured man. Steve directed the traffic to keep me and the unconscious man safe. Steve said he could hear me talking non-stop, saying all the appropriate words, as I knelt in the injured man's blood and stroked him gently. From my point of view, I was also having a conversation with the *spirit* of the man, trying to keep him calm and explain what was happening. I knew he was going to pass over so I tried to prepare him as he was obviously in shock. He told me his full name, age, where he worked, and even mentioned his estranged daughter. I, automatically relayed this 'accurate' information to the emergency crew when they arrived. The man died peacefully in hospital later the next day. The information I'd passed on to them was correct.

I did continue to explore my 'mediumship' and teach it to others in a sensible, evidence-based way. I was even invited to work with Glyn Edwards, CSNU at Arthur Findlay College, Stansted. After his sudden illness in 2003, Glyn visited us in our home in the Welsh hills. He received some private training and healing from us, which he felt he needed at that time. Over the years we

191

have met and worked alongside many international mediums as we continued to research, understand and challenge the practice.

We adopted several family mottos and I am sure, at times, our children got fed up of hearing them:

'Believe in yourself and everything is possible'

'A life lived in fear is a life half lived'

'Life is for living and meant to be fun'

'We just... get on with it!'

Over the years many friends have, temporarily, moved in with us. I am sure they, as well as the initially embarrassed teenage friends of our children, will remember our mealtime ritual. At the end of the meal I would ask each person to come up with three things that they have appreciated about that day. For example, I might say,

"Today, I appreciated the beautiful sunrise, the tasty curry Steve cooked – my favourite – and... I appreciate – I love my soft, velour purple dressing gown that always makes me feel comfy and warm."

Next, each person mentions three people or pets who they 'value' and why. For example,

"Today, I value the dog for making me smile when he balances the tennis ball on his nose, Sam (a friend) who made me laugh so much when we were planning Renate's birthday party, and a stranger who gave me some small change when I had none in the car park."

Our journey as healers has continued post cancer. I have studied psychology at PhD level, hold many Diplomas in various complementary therapies and an Advanced Diploma in Nutrition. Steve, my dad and I all became qualified SNU Spiritual Healers. Today, I am continuing my research in the field of Epigenetics.

We also continue to work with spiritually focused groups both in the UK and abroad – supporting each other on our journey through life. Striving to help others in their self-development has been a key factor that has consistently flowed through our work, home and spiritual life.

What did we both learn from that experience and episode in your lives?

The power of the mind is stronger than the body – mind over matter. It *is* possible to turn around a life threatening illness and death sentence. We can change things by the power of the mind, intent, will and desire.

Spirit is a reality. It highlighted for me my innate belief that we are a spirit in a body and we can, and do, manifest certain experiences in our lives.

193

We learned that healing assistance can come from, not only medical professions, but also from metaphysical means, for example via spiritual healers.

Over the years, research studies and reports have given scientific and medical explanations as to why Steve's method of survival worked. We were working on gut instinct and an inner knowing or belief that we were doing the right things to help Steve repair and renew his body.

Whatever the reader believes regarding the above, Steve and I hope you will not disregard the overall message within *Nipples to Kneecaps – to die or not to die with cancer* – of inspiration and hope in the face of great challenges. If you are given a diagnosis of cancer – in the past, present or in the future – I hope that that you will remember our story and still use and adapt our plan to help you manifest in your life the outcomes that you want. A cancer journey can be viewed as painful, frightening, unfair and terrible, but you can take another perspective and find the 'silver linings' and, as a result, feel more powerful than you ever felt have before. If one person can do it, so can you!

Defeat Cancer PLAN

1. Decide to take back control of your body, mind and spirit. Follow your own plan with focus, intent and passion.

2. Positivity culture: cultivate and keep a positive attitude in the home – no tears, no negativity, and no self-pity.
   a. Do not watch the news on TV (as it can be so negative) or any sad, depressing, negative programmes and films – be selective, ask yourself, "Will this make me smile or feel better about myself and the world?"
   b. Continually replace negative statements with positive statements. If a negative one comes out of your mouth or someone else's, say out loud or in your head a positive one – with conviction e.g. replace "I feel so ill" with "I will feel better tomorrow."
   c. Delete words like 'Can't', 'Impossible' and 'It's too difficult' from your vocabulary and replace them with their positive opposites or alternatives.

3. Laughter: laugh everyday – watch comedy shows, films, DVDs (at least one hour a day). Read jokes, funny books. Tell jokes, puns, and funny stories. Look for the 'funny side of life'. Spend time with people who make you laugh. What makes you laugh? Do that!

4. Visualisation: see the 'healing happen'. Visualise the cancer being destroyed and decide a way for it to leave your body. Visualise yourself as

whole and healthy, and doing things in the future that you enjoy. Keep focused and perform with passion.

5. Healing Mantra: "Tomorrow I will feel better. I am getting better every day." Although, it is always best to say things in the present tense, e.g. "I am healthy" – I have found some cancer patients feel this is too difficult – until they start to 'feel' an improvement. A useful mantra, introduced to me recently by Lucy Johnson, is "I am positively expecting great results no matter what I currently see before me. The universe is rearranging itself in my best interest right now." Repeat your mantra with focused intent at least three times every morning and night before you go to sleep.

6. The Healing Minute: join with healers in over 95 countries around the world in the healing minute. Send or receive healing energy at 10.00 and 22.00 your local time every day.

7. Complementary healing: receive complementary healing of your choice several times a week. Choose whichever helps you get into a meditative state (relaxed, peaceful) and results in you feeling refreshed, recharged, and more positive afterwards. We have found 'hands-on healing spiritual healing' (usually offered free in Spiritualist churches), aromatherapy massage, sound healing, reflexology, hot stone massage,

reiki, guided path workings/meditations etc. to be effective. Try these and others (too numerous to mention) to find which ones you like best.

8. Increase your knowledge: read books and watch videos related to naturopathic healing, healing therapies, mindest, positivity, e.g. TED talks, What the Bleep, the Placebo Effect, Truth About Cancer, Epigenetics. You may not agree with everything you see or hear (we didn't), but the point is that it is worth expanding your mind to consider the topics and points they raise.

9. Contemplate: who or what are you? Are you an eternal spirit in a body? Are you energy? What is your life force? Whenever life gets over-whelming or I have too many choices or I get stressed I sit still and repeat to myself, 'I am Spirit' 'I am at great peace within.'

10. Decide on the three most important things: you want to be, do or become in the future. Say them out loud to someone and have them at the back of your mind above all else. 'Believe in yourself and everything is possible!'

11. Side effects – positive spin: every time you are sick or experience a negative reaction related to any treatment, turn it into a positive, e.g. "There goes some more of the cancer!"

197

12. Energy: ask family and friends to pray, send healing energy, light a candle for you or whenever they think of you to imagine you healthy and well doing your favourite sport or activity – all positive energy directed your way will be welcome.

13. Live life: take steps to keep engaged in life and family/friend activities. Start a new hobby if necessary. The online chat groups and interactive games can be a lifeline to some.

14. Nature: go outside and connect to nature (daily if possible), even if it is only into your own garden. Breathe in the air, the smells, take in the whole experience with all your senses.

15. Keep going: the 'just get on with it' attitude. If people ask how you are, say, "I'm fine/good" rather than reliving all the treatment process, pains, worries etc.

16. Music: choose music that uplifts, energises and makes you happy.

17. Your words: think about how the words we say affected Emoto's crystals and water.

Appendix

The Healing Minute

"The Healing Minute takes place twice daily – at 10am and 10pm.

Every day people in 95 countries around the world join with the Sanctuary to focus their thoughts on healing for those in need and for world peace.

"We invite you to join us at 10 o'clock your own local time and add your own positive thought in a minute of meditation in sending energy to those in need wherever they are in the world and become part of a world energy peace force."
https://www.harryedwardshealingsanctary.org.uk/healingminute.html

Research Studies and Books

Epigenetics

1. Epigenetics is the science which explains how our environment (what we eat, drink, breathe, touch, think and perceive to be true) can turn our genes on/off. Research started to filter to the general public in the mid-nineties.
I now have an extensive library of books on Epigenetics, so I have only listed the first two which I read.

a. *Epigenetics: The Death of the Genetic Theory of Disease Transmission* by Joel Wallach

b. *The Epigenetics Revolution: How Modern Biology Is Rewriting Our Genetics, Disease and Inheritance* by Nessa Carey

2. We are not just our DNA – see the studies on twins.

> "Because identical twins develop from a single fertilized egg, they have the same genome. So any differences between twins are due to their environments, not genetics. Recent studies have shown that many environmentally induced differences are reflected in the epigenome."
> http://learn.genetics.utah.edu/content/epigenetics/twins/
> http://learn.genetics.utah.edu/content/epigenetics/

3. In simplified terms, epigenetics is the study of biological mechanisms (chemical reactions and the factors that influence them) that will switch genes on and off. It has been muted by some to be the 'future of medicine'.

Epigenetics Controls Genes. Certain circumstances in life can cause genes to be silenced or expressed over time. In other words, they can be turned off (becoming dormant) or turned on (becoming active).

Epigenetics Is Everywhere. What you eat, where you live, who you interact with, when you sleep, how you exercise, even aging – all of these can eventually cause chemical modifications around the genes that will turn those genes on or off over time. Additionally, in certain diseases such as cancer or Alzheimer's, various genes will be switched into the opposite state, away from the normal/healthy state.

Epigenetics Is Reversible. With 20,000+ genes, what will be the result of the different combinations of genes being turned on or off? The possible permutations are enormous! But if we could map every single cause and effect of the different combinations, and if we could reverse the gene's state to keep the good while eliminating the bad… then we could theoretically cure cancer, slow aging, stop obesity, and so much more."
http://www.whatisepigenetics.com/fundamentals/
https://www.facebook.com/epigeneticscoaching/
http://www.epigeneticscoach.com

Cells & Neuropeptides

1. In 1985, research by neuropharmacologist Candace Pert revealed that neuropeptide-specific receptors are present on the cell walls of both the brain and the immune system. This showed their close association with emotions and suggested mechanisms through which emotions and immunology are deeply interdependent. Negative thoughts manifest into chemical reactions that can impact the body by bringing more stress into the system and decreasing its immunity. In contrast, positive thoughts and emotions trigger neurochemical changes that reduce the immunosuppressive effects of stress.

2. *What the Bleep* is one of my favourite films – part documentary, part story. It employs animations to realize the radical knowledge that modern science (2004) has unearthed in recent years, in particular quantum physics. Powerful cinematic sequences explore the inner workings of the human brain. Quirky animation introduces us to the smallest form of consciousness in the body – the cell. Hilarious, in parts, and unforgettable. http://www.whatthebleep.com/

3. In 1994 Masaru Emoto froze water samples to observe them under a microscope. He was hoping to discover hexagonal crystals similar to snowflakes. From tap water he could not get any beautiful crystals, nor from rivers and lakes near big cities, but from those rivers and lakes kept

well away from developments did he observe amazingly beautiful crystals. Taking this further he observed the crystals of frozen distilled water after showing each sample certain words, different pictures, playing of diverse music and even praying over the water. The resulting photographs are breathtaking and thought provoking. Compare the 'Love/Appreciation' and 'Beautiful' crystals to 'You make me sick/I will kill you' and 'You Fool' crystals; compare a heavy metal song to Edelweiss, compare the crystals taken before and after the Buddhist prayer ceremony at Fujiwara dam.

It's worth considering that if the words we say, the music we hear, prayer and what we see can affect the cell structure of a water crystal in a test tube what happens to us (70% water) and our unborn children (a fertilised egg is 95% water) – inside? At any one moment 'our environment' and words are making beautiful crystals or ugly ones. I know which type I'd like to be creating in other people and children.
The Hidden Messages in Water by Masaru Emoto 5 Dec 2005

Placebo

You Are the PLACEBO Making Your Mind Matter by Dr. Joe Dispenza

Is it possible to heal by thought alone – without drugs or surgery? The truth is that it happens more often than you might expect…

"The key is making your inner thoughts more real than the outer environment, because then the brain won't know the difference between the two and will change to look as if the event has taken place. If you're able to do this successfully enough times, you'll transform your body and begin to signal new genes in new ways, producing epigenetic changes – just as though the imagined future event were real."

Laughter

1. *Anatomy of an Illness as Perceived by the Patient: Reflections on Healing and Regeneration* by Norman Cousins

2. *Ottawa lodges add humour to armamentarium in fight against cancer* CMAJ. 1990 Jan B Trent 2003 Mar https://www.ncbi.nlm.nih.gov/pmc/articles/PMC1451723

3. *The effect of mirthful laughter on stress and natural killer cell activity* Bennett MP[1], Zeller JM, Rosenberg L, McCann J.

"Laughter may reduce stress and improve NK cell activity. As low NK cell activity is linked to decreased disease resistance and increased morbidity in persons with cancer and HIV disease, laughter may be a useful cognitive-behavioral intervention."
https://www.ncbi.nlm.nih.gov/pubmed/12652882

4. *Social laughter is correlated with an elevated pain threshold* R. I. M. Dunbar, Rebecca Baron, Anna Frangou, Eiluned Pearce, Edwin J. C. van Leeuwen, Julie Stow, Giselle Partridge, Ian MacDonald, Vincent Barra, Mark van Vugt Published 14 September 2011.

"The results show that pain thresholds are significantly higher after laughter than in the control condition. This pain-tolerance effect is due to laughter itself and not simply due to a change in positive affect. We suggest that laughter, through an endorphin-mediated opiate effect, may play a crucial role in social bonding."
http://rspb.royalsocietypublishing.org/content/279/1731/1161

Laughter helps us to relax by shutting off a valve that transports stress and adrenaline throughout the body. Laughter helps combat stress by increasing blood flow throughout the body, boosts the immune system, heightens your threshold for pain and even assists in facilitating better breathing. The boost in blood flow helps break down blockages in arteries caused by stress and anxiety, releasing an uptick of T-cells, B-cells and Gamma-interferons – cells and proteins that fight against disease.

"A merry heart does good like a medicine, but a broken spirit dries the bones." (Proverbs 17:22)

Mindset

1. *The Lazy Man's Way to Riches: Dyna/Psyc can give you everything in the world you really want!* by Joe Karbo (1973)

2. New scientific discoveries about the biochemical effects of the brains functioning show that all the cells in your body are affected by your thoughts. Bruce H. Lipton, Ph.D., a renowned cell biologist describes the precise molecular pathways through which this occurs. https://www.brucelipton.com/books/biology-of-belief

Meditation

1. *Mindfulness-based cancer recovery and supportive-expressive therapy maintain telomere*

length relative to controls in distressed breast cancer survivors

> Linda E. Carlson PhD, Tara L. Beattie PhD, Janine Giese-Davis PhD, Peter Faris PhD, Rie Tamagawa PhD, Laura J. Fick PhD, Erin S. Degelman MSc, Michael Speca PsyD
> First published: 3 November 2014
> World-First Evidence Suggests That Meditation Alters Cancer Survivors' Cells.
>
> For the first time, scientists have found clear biological evidence that meditation and support groups can affect us on a cellular level.

2. *Interaction between Neuroanatomical and Psychological Changes after Mindfulness-Based Training* Emiliano Santarnecchi, Sicilia D'Arista, Eutizio Egiziano, Concetta Gardi, Roberta Petrosino, Giampaolo Vatti, Mario Reda, Alessandro Rossi

> Published: October 20, 2014
> Italian scientists also showed that mindfulness training can change the structure of our brains.

1. *Healing the Heart: Integrating Complementary Therapies and Healing Practices Into the Care of Cardiovascular Patients* Mary Jo Kreitzer, PhD, RN; Mariah Snyder, PhD, RN

> "Complementary therapies and healing practices have been found to reduce stress, anxiety and lifestyle patterns known to contribute to cardiovascular disease. Promising therapies include imagery and hypnosis, meditation, yoga, tai chi, prayer, music, exercise, diet and use of dietary supplements"

> "Complementary therapies have been a key component of nursing practice – both the administration of specific therapies and the underlying holistic philosophy."
> http://www.ahc.umn.edu/img/assets/7444/healheart.pdf

2. *Developing an integrative therapies in primary care program.* Anastasi JK, Capili B, Schenkman F. Nurse Educ. 2009 Nov

Nature

1. *A forest bathing trip increases human natural killer activity and expression of anti-cancer proteins in female subjects.* Li Q[1], Morimoto K, Kobayashi M, Inagaki H, Katsumata M, Hirata Y, Hirata K, Shimizu T, Li YJ, Wakayama Y, Kawada T, Ohira T, Takayama N, Kagawa T, Miyazaki Y. 2007

2. *Visiting a forest, but not a city, increases human natural killer activity and expression of anti-cancer proteins.* Li Q[1], Morimoto K, Kobayashi M, Inagaki H, Katsumata M, Hirata Y, Hirata K, Suzuki H, Li YJ, Wakayama Y, Kawada T, Park BJ, Ohira T, Matsui N, Kagawa T, Miyazaki Y, Krensky AM. 2008

3. *Healthy nature healthy people: 'contact with nature' as an upstream health promotion intervention for populations* Cecily Maller, Mardie Townsend, Anita Pryor, Peter Brown, Lawrence St Leger 2005

Jacuzzi of Despair

http://metro.co.uk/2016/11/02/theres-a-jacuzzi-of-des-pair-in-the-sea-and-if-you-go-in-you-die-6230503/

A deadly pool of toxic chemicals which researchers have called 'the Jacuzzi of Despair' sits on the sea floor 3,000 below the Gulf of Mexico.

The strange pool of brine and chemicals kills animals unlucky enough to fall in, with toxic chemicals spewing out like an undersea waterfall – with its edges littered with dead crabs.

In culture of positivity, I would prefer you to focus on the hydrothermal vents, chemosynthesis and 100s of new species discovered in the dark at the bottom of the sea.

http://ocean.si.edu/ocean-videos/hydrothermal-vent-creatures

Comedies 1980s

Blazing Saddles Fawlty Towers Airplane The Comic Strip	The Young Ones Ever Decreasing Circles The Fall and Rise of Reginald Perrin	Are You Being Served? Smith and Jones Black Adder
The Good Life Taxi Cheers The Two Ronnies	The Lenny Henry Show Monty Python's Flying Circus Some Mothers Do 'Av 'Em	Spitting Image Porridge The Goodies Open All Hours
Allo! Allo! Dad's Army	Any spaghetti western Not the Nine O'clock News	Comedy Club Rising Damp

Thanks

I want to list all of you who have contributed, encouraged or helped us in some way, but that would fill another book! I want to shout out to the world in thanks and recognition of all the names of every single wonderful supportive person (including you!) who lived the journey with us at the time or since. So please know that you ALL mean so much us, that we appreciate and value you even if we have never met in person. Thank you also to those who helped and supported me in the writing process.

Having resisted to list names, please forgive me though as I now single out one person – Steve Brown. My soul mate, lover, partner and supporter. Thank you, thank you, thank you for being you and for 'growing old' with me!

Thank you to all my readers. Your opinion will help others decide if they want to purchase my book. If you enjoyed this book, please consider leaving an honest review on the site where you purchased it. Thank you. Want to find out about what I am working on next? Sign up on my website and keep updated on the latest news.

https://www.nipplestokneecaps.com

New Books Coming Soon by Mandy Brown

Bonegirl – a supernatural, shamanic story for the younger reader about how a young girl finds her own power to defeat the Scanlon Hunters, her bullies at school.

The Missing Magical Mindset – the missing secrets and techniques to achieving your dreams in life.

Focus on Mediumship – step by step guide to understanding and developing your psychic and mediumistic abilities.

He'll Never Talk – a true inspirational story about the struggles and triumphs of a deafblind child and his family.

Contact

Contact Mandy & Steve with your queries about the book content, any questions you may have and to request us for Speaker bookings.

Email: mandybrownauthor@gmail.com
Website: http://www.nippletokneecaps.com
Facebook: https://www.facebook.com/mandybrownauthor/

Printed in Great Britain
by Amazon